KETO DIET

FOR WOMEN OVER 50

Learn the Healthiest Ketogenic Habits and Recipes for Beginners That Will Make You Lose Weight Fast and Restore Your Metabolism to Regain Your Confidence

Melissa Moore

© Copyright 2021 - All rights reserved.

Table of Contents

CHAPTER 1:

What is the Ketogenic Diet?

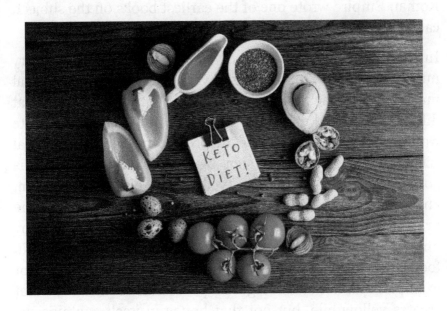

Any diet is more than what meets the eye. It is in short, the potential of a lifestyle. What we eat everyday goes hand in hand with our attitudes, beliefs and ways of being. Picking the right diet must then align with these aspects of lifestyle and vice versa. For a diet to be successful, it must reflect the beliefs, lifestyle choices and attitudes of the dieter. Many times this will require a radical change in the way we view food, and what we come to expect from it.

The tradition of diets goes back to ancient human history, where we ate whatever we could find. Then with the rise of civilizations came the use of agriculture, livestock and newer methods for producing foodstuffs. Everyone knew food for what it was—energy. The same stuff that took us from a state of hunger to a state of fullness. Those who did not eat because of famine or disease paid the ultimate price. But it wasn't until much later that there was higher interest in the what food consisted of. Galen, a renowned ancient physician of the Roman Empire wrote one of the earliest books on the subject, called *The Properties of Foodstuffs.*

In *The Properties of Foodstuffs* Galen talks about rudimentary nutrition, and how food affects physiological and psychological makeup. Even back then (circa 100 A.D.) physicians knew that different food had different properties. But what Galen wrote would mostly go on to be disproved by modern natural sciences. For example, Galen believed that the body was governed by the four humors (yellow bile, black bile, phlegm, and blood). Any imbalance in these four humors was the primary cause of disease. While Galen didn't say that eating any one food produced any of the humors, he did say that certain foods influenced the creation of such humors. He believed, for example, that honey undergoes a process inside the body that creates yellow bile, but not that honey in itself contains the humor.

How Galen came to such conclusions is not clear, but there is some evidence from the ancient world that suggests a connection between sugar and disease. Diabetes when first observed by ancient Greek and Egyptian physicians was manifested by a sweetening of the urine. In fact, the technical term for the various types of diabetes is called *diabetes mellitus,* diabetes meaning to siphon and mellitus meaning "honey" or "sweet". It comes from the fact that physicians observed the urine to be sweet (and probably yellowish) to resemble honey. There is a connection here between Galen's belief that a imbalance in the humors caused diseases, and that sugar was present in the urine of diabetics. By eating too much honey (sugar) one would unbalance the four humors, thus resulting in disease. Of course back then physicians really had no idea what diabetes was, or how to properly treat it.

But it was essentially that a foodstuff could potentially cause disease. Even if Galen's theory of humors was woefully incorrect, it still hinted at a modern phenomenon of the affects of food consumption. Namely, that certain foods cause certain biochemical reactions inside the body. These reactions then go on to form changes in our physiological and psychological makeup. So Galen wasn't that wrong after all.

The diet—or what we eat—quickly become a matter of medicine as much as a matter of home economics. Physicians routinely prescribed food as a possible therapy for. Don't eat this, eat that instead. Limit consumption of this food, and so on. We know now that diet and disease go hand in hand. Cardiovascular disease, diabetes, even cancer are affected to some degree by the things that we eat. Galen knew this, but was unable to produce the necessary scientific reasoning behind it. Today we have modern science, biochemistry and loads of experimental data that proves, once and for all, that we are what we eat.

In the tradition of using diet to treat certain ailments, physicians in the 19th and 20th centuries tried treating some of their patients with food. Obesity, for example, was hardly ever observed before the 19th century when industrialization really took off. New milling techniques for separating the germ from the endosperm of wheat resulted into new varieties of wheat being manufactured. This wheat was fattening, because it was refined from much of the natural properties found in whole grain. For the first time in industrialized nations, people started getting fat. And it wasn't just the kings or people from affluence who gained corpulent bodies. Even common folk were getting fat.

It is around this time that the first low-carbohydrate diets were being experimented with. Something about refined grain—and the products made from it—was causing a stir. We all know that bread tends to make us fat, especially if eaten in conjunction with sugar or other refined foods. Physicians were being asked by their patients how they could slim down in their weight. Somewhere along the way, the wisdom of Galen was lost, and those same patients who were considered "corpulent" were told to stop eating so much. It wasn't that the properties of food were making them fat, but that their own self-control was the problem. These people were in a sense, digging their own grave by eating more than their fair share.

Low-Carb Revolution

During the first half of the 19th century there was a race for the cure of diabetes. Or at least, for a competent therapy. Up to that point, diabetes was a deadly disease with few, if any, existing medications. The discovery of insulin by Sir Frederick Banting in 1921 marked a pivotal point in the development of diabetes treatments. Later, diabetes was classified into two distinct diseases, type 1 and type 1 diabetes. But even before insulin was discovered, diets were being used to treat it. The most effective type of diet for its treatment was the low-carb variety.

This is around the time that the modem ketogenic diet was discovered. It is essentially a low-carb, high-fat diet with enough protein to sustain muscle growth and repair. During the 1920's this type of diet was used to great success for treating epilepsy in young children. Before medication existed that helped control the convulsions of a epileptic fit, physicians observed that eliminating grains, starchy fruits, and starchy vegetables from the diet resulted in lesser convulsions. The keto diet would go on to be used to treat other neurological disorders like Alzheimer's, brain tumors, and Parkinson's in conjunction with modern therapies.

The keto diet derives its name from ketosis, a process in which the body directly converts fat into usable energy. In 1921 a physician named Rollin Turner Woodyatt observed the existence of compounds named *beta*-Hydroxybutyric acid, acetoacetate, and acetone in the liver of those who were either starving or following a low-carb diet for diabetes. Today they are recognized as some of the "ketone bodies" or ketones that the liver produces to metabolize fat as energy. Later, physician Dr. Russell Morse Wilder working for the Mayo Clinic would first use the term "ketogenic diet" to describe a low-carb, high fat diet that produced these ketone bodies. He would treat his epilepsy patients with such a diet, making it the first time the ketogenic diet was used to treat it. The rest as they say, is history.

You have probably heard about keto in just about every online publication and social media website. There is a resurgence going on of the diet, with top celebrities using it as well as fitness gurus the world over. Keto is touted as being excellent for weight loss, meanwhile having adequate protein content to stimulate muscle growth. Best of all, it keeps that weight down by putting you in a perpetual state of ketosis. Keto may even be used to help treat obesity and diabetes by some accounts. Others say that they have completely given up buying expensive diabetes medication because a keto diet helps them regulate blood sugar levels just as well.

Above all, keto is a lifestyle. It means making healthier choices at the grocery store and coming home with nothing but the freshest, whole foods ingredients. Unlike other diets, keto doesn't make a compromise between taste and nutrition. Every meal is based around either a high-fat or protein component. You aren't allowed to eat most carbohydrate foods, but there are plenty of other options available to fill in calories. Keto, being a whole food diet, also prohibits the consumption of processed foods. Together the whole food and low-carbohydrate philosophy contribute to an incredibly healthy and sustainable lifestyle. You will feel better while staying fit at the same time.

Why choose low-carb?

Once upon a time, carbohydrates were considered the number one food source. If you looked into the office of any pediatrician or peeked inside an American school cafeteria in the 90's to early 2000's you would see reproductions of the food pyramid. Back then, the bottom row or the base of the pyramid was made up of grains and starches. Cereals, pastas and breads formed the basis of the recommended American diet. Modern reproductions of the same pyramid now have water as the base, and carbohydrates have lesser importance.

This is no doubt attributed to the spiking rise in obesity and type 2 diabetes rates. Carbohydrates, unlike fats and proteins, cause us to more readily gain weight. Low-carb diets get rid of these foods because they aren't really necessary for bodily function (ketosis can play the same role that carbohydrates do) and because they make us fat.

Low-carb diets were born from the same observations in the 18th century that industrialization was creating more food than ever before, and that processed and refined grains resulted in weight gain. Food manufacturing or the creation of processed food products, coincided with a rise in average weight gain. Today, processed foods are out of control. Virtually anything that we eat has a complex production cycle that involves both mechanical and chemical means. Ingredients lists are longer than ever. And even then, the manufacturer doesn't always tell you what an ingredient means or how it was used in the production cycle.

Eating too much carbohydrates is easy. A single apple might give you upwards to 25g of carbs. It doesn't help that carbs taste good and make us feel good. Of all the foods out there, carbs are most cited as foods of relaxation. But too much of a good thing can be bad. Nobody doubts that eating too much cake or junk food is bad for them. And yet, they still do it, because they get a pleasurable response from it.

The two main ingredients that fuel weight gain in these type of foods are sugar, and refined carbohydrates. Both of these act like a conduit for weight gain. They tend to be calorically dense, and not filling at all. Eating them satisfies you for a few hours, but you are always hungry afterwards. Once sugar or a carb enters the body, it must either be used as energy or it will get stored for later as fat cells. Most of us will not burn all of the calories that we consume in a given day. Keeping track of daily calorie requirements is already difficult enough, and throwing in sugary or highly refined carbohydrates makes it even harder.

These foods are easy to spot: anything that contains sugar is likely to be a refined carb, because sugar is a type of refined carb. Next, anything that is made out of a refined product, like refined grain is also a refined carb. Any food that combines both refined white flour and refined sugar is among the worst things you can eat. Next come the endless list of processed foods. These include sugary foods like sodas, sugary beverages, candies, and other confectioneries usually sold in packaging.

Eating a healthy diet while still having a high carbohydrate output is possible, but unsustainable for the average person. For centuries ancient and indigenous societies subsisted on a few, high carbohydrate staple foods like rice and starchy vegetables without exhibiting large obesity or type 2 diabetes rates among the population. The simple reason for this is that those foods are still considered whole, contain little to no sugar, and are unrefined. Another contributing factor is that these societies tend to eat at their caloric requirements. They tend to be active, rather than sedentary, and their relationship with food is vastly different from ours.

For the average consumer, eating a healthy high carbohydrate diet is much more difficult. Processed foods are high in added sugars and other extra ingredients. Refined foods are easy to manufacture and store, generally sell well, and are ubiquitous on the market floor. Someone looking to lose weight is better of cutting out carbohydrates all together and sticking with a whole foods, ketogenic diet.

The problem with sugar

Sugar is a general term used to describe a wide range of sweet tasting carbohydrates. In particular, they are called saccharides. Most of them are derived from the sugar found in fruits and vegetables. Table sugar (sucrose) comes from beets, canes and other sources. Fructose, another type of sugar is found in fruits. It is what gives fruits such as apples and watermelon such high carbohydrate content. Separating the pure sugar molecule from the whole food is done by a refining process. That is, sugar never reaches such high quantities in the natural world. At least not if you are eating within well portioned sizes. In contrast, the refined product may be used in food items that are over saturated with sugar. Think coca cola, and the endless list of brands for fruit juice.

The problem with sugar is multifold. It is good tasting, making it potentially addictive and pleasurable to eat. Your brain gets a pleasure response, telling it that eating sugar is good. Sugar is also a type of refined carb, meaning that they cause weight gain. Food companies know that humans have a sweet tooth, which is unfortunately taken advantage of for profit. Snacks for children are loaded with sugar, for example. And food labels never have a warning that sugar can lead to diabetes and obesity, despite the fact that both diseases have reached epidemic levels in the United States. Sugar is calorically dense and offers little nutritional value. It ramps up calorie intake quickly, and may then get turned into fat if it upsets the balance of calories in and calories out.

Perhaps most upsetting, sugar is everywhere. It lurks under different ingredient names like sucralose, dextrose, high-fructose corn syrup, and so on. Processed foods will regularly use some form of sweetener or preservative that are sugar based. This makes it increasingly difficult to "eat clean". Everything from baked good, crackers, so called "healthy" drinks, and even processed sandwich meats may contain sugar. In recent years the prevalence of sugar in the food industry has led to some health conscious organizations to push for a "sugar tax", which is already making inroads in many. jurisdictions. Some countries like the UK have already adopted it at the federal level.

Sugar in a way, is toxic to the body. This is evident in the rise of type 2 diabetes, a condition characterized by high elevations of sugar (glucose) in the blood. The same sugar molecules in the bloodstream bind into proteins, creating new compounds called Advanced Glycation End Products (AGE's). It is a fitting acronym, because what these compounds do is accelerate the creation of wrinkles in the skin, sagging eyes, and so on. The same AGE's may be responsible for causing damage to blood vessels and organs in diabetics.

In short, long-term sugar consumption accelerates the aging process. This is true not only for the physical characteristics of aging, like wrinkly skin and weight gain, but also some of the physiological characteristics as well. High consumption of refined carbohydrates is associated with inflammation inside th body. Carbonated sugar drinks are associated with accelerated bone density loss (osteoporosis). And many diabetics suffer from lower immunity because of the high sugar in their blood.

How keto can help

The standard ketogenic diet allows for very little in terms of carbohydrates and sugar. A formal definition of keto is a diet that is high in fat and low in carbohydrates, which are universally of the unrefined variety. This means that table sugar is obviously out of the equation. Other forms of sugar like the fructose in fruit can be occasionally enjoyed. But note that fructose is still derived from a "whole food". You aren't going to find apples and pears inside of boxes at your grocery store with a long list of ingredients, for example. Adopting a ketogenic lifestyle can slowly wean your body of it's sugar and refined carbohydrate dependency by putting you in a constant state of ketosis. Doing so will slowly reverse the effects of sugar toxicity on your body, and ultimately help you burn off fat that is simply sugar stored for the long run.

Staying in ketosis is simple: eating a diet that is low in carbohydrates will force your body to burn fat instead. Note that most of the carbs that you do eat in a keto diet (usually less than 50g or even 25g a day) will come from non-starchy vegetables. These are your leafy greens, your spinach, lettuce, kale and celery. Technically, all forms of vegetables are carbohydrate. But their carbohydrate content is dictated by whether they are starchy or non-starchy. Something that is starchy like a white potato is loaded with carbs, and are not allowed on keto. Other alternatives, like sweet potato, are lower in carbohydrates and may be used a substitute.

Over time, your sugar cravings may even go away entirely. People who follow strict keto diets end up craving fat, of all things. These come in the form of healthy fats, found in food items like dairy products, olive and coconut oil, nuts, fatty cuts of meat and fish, creams and so forth. Craving fat isn't a bad thing necessarily. It is by and large, a better alternative than craving sugar.

How to gauge your overall heath

Someone's health goes beyond simply taking note of their physical fitness. It also covers a wide range of psychological markers. How you feel on a daily basis is also very important. Someone who is constantly bloated, suffering from low-energy or mood swings probably isn't all that healthy. The same can be said for the individual who isn't getting enough sleep. These factors and many more all contribute to a singular thing called lifestyle. A lifestyle will be shaped by many things, including attitudes, beliefs, personal circumstance and so on. A lifestyle is also influenced by the choices that we make. Someone born with type a diabetes didn't have a choice. Someone who developed type 2 diabetes after years of eating a diet high in refined carbs did have a choice. Philosophy of freedom of choice and sugar addictions set aside, anyone has the power to change their lifestyle given enough effort.

When it comes to determine physical fitness and health, there is a standard formula to follow. Weight in relation to height is a standard indicator used to measure body composition, or how much fat a person is. This of course, the body-mass index(BMI), which is used as the first line diagnostic for obesity. A high BMI indicates a high concentration of fat. While the BMI isn't perfect, it works for most people. A body builder or Olympic weightlifting may have a high BMI, but may still be perfectly healthy for example. Calculating BMI is trivially easy. It is a simply equation of weight in kilograms over height in meters squared. There are many calculators on the web that can help you find your BMI.

Next is the diet. What types of food are you eating on a daily basis, and how much of it? And are your daily calories exceeding your daily calories burned? How many calories you need will depend on your age, weight, gender and level of physical activity. Women tend to need less calories than men, all other factors being equal. Elderly and younger than adolescent children also require less caloric energy. Finally, those with sedentary lifestyles and desk jobs need less calories than laborers and physically active people. Calculators exist for finding out your calorie needs as well. What you are looking for is an approximation of your basal metabolic rate (BMR) which tells you, more or less, how many calories your body burns without you doing anything.

Someone who is "fit" has an average, or near average BMI, and a varied diet that is at or slightly above or below their BMR. But the more those measures stray from the average, the more likely that the person is unhealthy, and that they make unhealthy lifestyle choices. Eating significantly above your BMR will inevitably cause weight gain. If the majority of those calories are derived from less than ideal food sources (refined carbohydrates, processed food, sugar) then you are also likely doing damage to your body through sugar toxicity, and are accelerating aging.

Here the ketogenic lifestyle offers a possible solution on the road to wellness. The whole foods approach allows you to eat satiating, all natural meals that keep you fuller for longer and make you less likely to eat above your calories. Furthermore, ketosis will help you burn stubborn body fat in the process. The keto diet is not for everyone, and tends to be one of the more "difficult" diets to complete. But if you play your cards right, eat the right things and monitor the way you feel on the diet, then you too can have success with the ketogenic lifestyle.

CHAPTER 2:

How Our Bodies Work

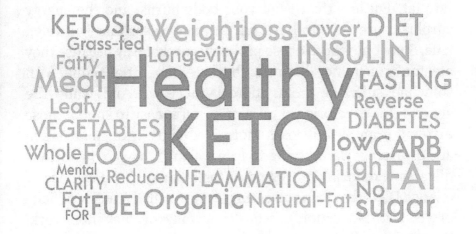

We know from Galen and from all of the physicians, biochemists and nutritionists that came after him that now two pieces of food are the same. This is true among food groups and true across them. A carbohydrate is vastly different from a protein. A starchy vegetable is vastly different from a non-starchy green. And like we also learned from Galen, it isn't necessarily that the food contains a certain property that alters our body, but that the processes of digestion inside our bodies interacts with the food's properties to bring about change. A simpler way to look at it is that the body is closed from the outside world. Once you put in foreign objects into your body, hundred of different levers, gears and switches go off in succession. This is the power of biochemistry inside us, choreographing a wicked dance of cells, hormones and nutrients.

The basis of weight gain

Weight gain is complicated. It will vary on a case by case basis in between individuals, but there are some general laws that seem to apply to everyone. The first, as you no doubt have heard by now, is the rule of calories in vs calories out. Eat more than your body burns, and the excess energy will get turned into fat. Eat less than what your body burns, and the energy surplus causes you to burn fat. In many cases that will reign true. Someone who is obese probably got that way because they ate too much, not because they ate too little. Same with someone suffering from anorexia nervous. And while the general rule of calories in vs calories out is easy to spot in those extreme examples, it loses more credibility with the average Joe or average Jane trying to lose weight. They go on various diets, try exercising more and so forth to usurp the balance of energy. Diets that focus on eating less are called "caloric deficit" or "caloric restriction" diets. They may or may not work. Restricting calories and exercising regularly still may or may not work.

The complexity comes from the distinct biophysical makeup of our bodies. No two body is alike. We all have different histories of metabolism, diet, and especially genetics that may play a role. Since nobody can really tell what is going on inside our bodies, it is difficult to generalize dieting advise. Large populations of like people tend to share the same ailments, risk-factors and other demographics. Asian countries, for example, were traditionally very lean compared to western nations. In recent years this has changed, with type 2 diabetes and obesity on the rise all over the globe. The Asian diet traditionally consist of the white rice staple food in conjunction with meat (especially sea food) and noodles. High in carbohydrates yes, but still they have traditional enjoyed smaller waist lines. In poorer areas of Asian countries this also reigns true.

So if our bodies are different, how can we reliably lose weight or create healthy habits for the long run? The ideal dieting advice will show results for a great many of people, and not just a select few. Or even the lucky few, who for whatever reason, a given diet will work for them but not for the other person. Another difficult arises in that these diets are hard to quantify uniformly. Scientific studies on diets are able to regulate food intake to a T (assuming the participants aren't cheating). But even so, sample sizes for these studies tend to be small, definitely lesser than the thousands, and so cannot be generalized for entire populations. Anecdotal dieting advice also doesn't work. Because two people can say the are following the same diet and yet have vastly different caloric intake and choices of food. Why? Because counting your macros, counting your calories, and making sure you don't over do it is a hard thing to do. Some may even say that doing so is impractical.

Properties of the macro nutrients

A good place to start is understanding why we gain weight in the first place. We eat some food, digest it, and then expel it. The nutrients or the stuff inside food are what determine everything. Most of the bulk of the food gets expelled as waste after the intestines have finished absorbing the nutrients fully. Whether a food is a protein, carbohydrate or fat it has the potential for causing weight gain. Every food is different, but they each have a value of energy attached to them called the calorie. You can probably imagine what would happen if you binged on any one of theses types of foods for too long.

Proteins are slow digesting, and fulling. When we eat at a barbecue or at a buffet, we get full quickly if we choose to eat mostly meat dishes. At some point, most of us will hit a "wall" during a meal where we cannot physically eat anymore, or doing so causes us significant effort. Eventually we do get hungry again, but it may be many hours afterwards. A large meal that is high in protein will go a long way. Note that being hungry or full doesn't really correlate to the caloric content of food, only how quickly it digests. Proteins in particular sent hormonal messages to the brain telling it to slow down on eating because the body requires extra work to digest them. On the whole, eating an excess of calories from protein alone is possible, but difficult.

Dietary fat is somewhere in between protein and carbohydrates in terms of filling factor. Fat is calorically denser than the other two macro nutrients. One gram of protein or carbs is equal to four calories. Meanwhile 1 gram of fat gives you roughly 9 calories. This is the 4-4-9 rule, and it generally holds true. But not all carbohydrate sources will conform to it. But it effectively means that on average, fat gives you more bang for your buck in terms of the bulk of food and energy derived from it. And again, binging on fat isn't something people are used to. Nobody is really chowing down bars of butter or drinking entire gallons of milk. Fat has more of an additive nature—it is used to fry foods, to season for taste and so on. In that case it is the combined nature of the food that is making you eat it. At the same barbecue or buffet from before they may be serving breaded fried chicken, buttered shrimp, Caesar salad with shreds of cheese and doused in marinade, and so forth. Many people starting up on the keto diet will find that getting enough fat into their diet is difficult.

Carbohydrates are an entirely different beast. And refined carbohydrates are like the apex predator of a skinny waist line. If we return to the buffet example, refined carbohydrates are capable of hijacking the fullness response you get from hormonal activity. Almost everyone, whether young or old, can make more room for dessert. When the ice cream platter comes our way, we instinctually unbutton our pants to let more in. This is because unlike fat or protein, we receive a major dopamine hit when we eat sugary or refined foods. This makes it exceeding easy to go beyond daily caloric requirements and to ignore the fact that our bodies are already full in a single meal. Carbohydrates are quick digesting foods, and their refined variety are like the nutritional equivalent of crack cocaine. They hit the bloodstream instantly, raising your blood sugar levels through the roof. And they don't really fill us up in the first place. The equivalent calories still enter your body, your brain just doesn't register it and creates a hunger response mere hours after a high carbohydrate meal.

What do you mean bread makes me fat?

Unlike the other two macro nutrients, carbohydrates directly impact the fat storage cycle. Sure, the other two do it to degree as well (calories in vs calories out) but carbohydrates are the only food that raise blood sugar or blood glucose levels. In case you slept through freshman biology class, our cells all need chemical energy to do the things that they do. This includes dividing, repairing themselves, and basically helping us stay alive. Each cell is like a well oiled machine that needs fuel to sustain activity. And the principle fuel of choice is glucose, or sugar.

There is nothing particularly interesting about glucose. It is found in our blood stream, and also in the table sugar that we eat. In this case, Galen was incorrect. Glucose is directly found inside of the food in the case of sugar, it doesn't need to be created by the body in that case. Carbohydrates are long chains of sugars or saccharides. Sucrose, the scientific name for the sugar we all know and love, is a disaccharide, meaning that it is made up of two distinct saccharides (sugar) molecules. These are one glucose, and one fructose. The fructose should be no surprise, as table sugar is derived from beets and sometimes sugarcane.

The body can directly use glucose, but not fructose. You increase the concentration of sugar in your blood by simply consuming the stuff. Other carbohydrates like bread, pasta and starchy vegetables are first converted into glucose. This is more of a Galenic scenario, where glucose needs to be derived from something, rather than directly accumulated in the blood stream. The fructose from table sugar, for example, needs to be also converted into glucose first by the liver. Once the glucose is free flowing in the blood, it can be delivered to whatever cell, organ or tissue that needs it. Our brains are notoriously glucose hungry. Some 20% of all available caloric energy will go to our noggins.

But once our cells have had their fill, the glucose isn't really needed. And since its already in the blood, it can't really be turned into waste and expelled. If it could, then obesity and type 2 diabetes would never be a thing. Some of the excess glucose will get turned into fat by the liver. It is sometimes called adipose tissue, which can either form underneath the skin (subcutaneous fat) or inside organs (visceral fat). This fat in turn, can be tapped into when glucose is in short supply. But with our modern diets, glucose is almost never in short supply. The fat never goes away. It just stays there. Caloric restriction and strenuous exercise may deplete glucose stores, causing this fat to eventually be melted down. But for the average Joe or Jane, burning this fat is incredibly difficult.

There is some reason to believe that eating a diet at the correct calorie requirements while still being high in refined carbs is bad for you. This makes intuitive sense, as you can eat a standard 2,000 calorie diet made up of junk food and still gain weight. Those who strongly believe in calories in vs calories out believe this is false. They believe that one can lose weight by simple eating at a caloric deficit. But not every calorie is creating equal. We know that the three macro nutrients are different, and that eating a majority of one type of macro will cause different effects in the body.

What is the deal with keto?

Many who are introduced to keto balk at the idea of eating a majority of calories from dietary fat. At some level, it is easy to confuse dietary fat for body fat or adipose tissue. There is a misconception that dietary fat literally makes you fat, but the truth is more nuanced than that. Dietary fat consists of oils, lipids and molecules called triglycerides. Fats contain more calories per gram on average than either proteins or cabs, making the a good candidate for weight gain from over eating. The calories in vs calories out school of thought tells us this much. Fats are fattening for the sole reason that they are dense in calories—it is easy to overeat with greasy, fatty foods, like pizza, fast food and so on. But there is difference between a whole foods diet and one that is necessarily greasy. Here again is the problem of fullness—your body only registers being full when it has consumed enough quantities of food bulk. Our bodies are dumb, and cannot easily tell when they had had enough calories. Since fats pack more calories into less food, we don't always get full from greasy meals, which is a good way to balloon in weight.

If you pay attention to nutritional science at all then you have probably heard a thing or two about cholesterol, especially in regards to fat. Things like eggs, bacon, red meat and so on are said to raise cholesterol. But in recent decades there has been many conflicting information on the subject. One doctor will say to limit egg yolk intake, and another will say that eggs are a healthy super food. Cholesterol is often scary to think about, because we all know that high cholesterol is associated with cardiovascular disease. These are your heart attacks and strokes, and nobody wants to willingly raise their chances of suffering from either. But what people consider even less, is that sugar can do the same thing. The majority of diabetes related fatalities are not due to organ or kidney failure, but to cardiovascular disease. This is because over time, high concentrations of glucose in the blood can calcify arteries, much in the same way that cholesterol can block them. The end result is largely the same—higher incidence of heart attack and stroke.

So which is worse for you, sugar or fat? Certainly, there have been campaigns in the past to paint dietary fat as public enemy #1. But the fat paranoia era only resulted in new products being conceived with the "low-fat" sticker on them. These low-fat varieties where invariably loaded with sugar to make up for it. It didn't really preset a solution to the perceived problem, as sugar is just as bad, if not worse, than cholesterol. Normalizing sugar consumption in lieu of dietary fat makes it seem like its okay to eat that low-fat yogurt or peanut butter or what have you, when the reality is that the sugar can lead to the same complications as cholesterol.

Not all cholesterol is bad in the first place. Normally we have small amounts of cholesterol in our cells that aid in the creation of hormones. Our bodies need cholesterol, but we can usually make enough on our own without needed any extra. Cholesterol generally comes in two different types: LDL or low-density proteins, the "bad" cholesterol that clogs arteries and HDL or high-density proteins which is sometimes regarded as the "good" cholesterol. HDL is good in the sense that it really isn't harmful to you. LDL is bad because too much of it puts you at risk for heart disease. There is also a third measure called total cholesterol which is a combination of both cholesterols in the blood. A high total cholesterol may be alarming to a doctor, especially when the ratios of LDL to HDL are high. This would mean that most of the cholesterol flowing in the blood is the bad variety.

Bad cholesterol is said to come from "unhealthy" fats these are your saturated and trans fats. Saturated fats are common in processed foods, fried foods, some dairy products and in vegetable oils. Trans fats appear on the same type of products, and were traditionally used to make margarine. Nowadays, trans fats are making a mass exit from the modern diet. They are harder to find on store shelves, as the general population has been hammered with information about how deadly they are. Many countries even ban them outright.

Even so, saturated fat is contained in many whole, and otherwise perfectly healthy food. By eliminating processed foods from the diet, you are already getting rid of the worst offenders of saturated fats anyways. Things like greasy fast food will be off the menu on the keto diet, as will ice cream, most chocolate, potato chips and candy. Another big offender are cured meats like salami, pepperoni and sand which meats. These two can be safely removed from the diet. Other foods that contain saturated fats and are okay to eat may include cheese, cream, butter, lard and coconut oil. Again, your diet won't be subsisting wholly on these foods at all. The other major source of saturated fat will be from animal proteins such as red meat. If cholesterol is a concern, you can elect to limit red meat consumption and use poultry or fish instead. Even among these options, none of them will be 100% saturated fat,

Other types of fat in the keto diet include mono unsaturated fats and polyunsaturated fats. Both of these fats are categorically better than the saturated variety and are healthy to eat. Mono saturated fats include things like avocados, olive oil, nuts and seeds and tallow. Polyunsaturated fats are found in fish, grass feed beef, eggs, and dairy sourced from grass fed cows. Note that dietary fat sources are composed of different types of fats. None will be wholly on type of saturated or unsaturated fat but have some combination thereof.

Going on keto doesn't immediately mean that your cholesterol will raise, but for many it is a concern. Those with existing high levels of cholesterol in particular should excise caution when going on the diet, and speak with their doctors beforehand. If cholesterol levels do rise during the diet, it may be prudent to cut back on fat sources or to forgo the diet altogether.

What about alcohol?

A common question that comes with keto diets is whether you can still enjoy your favorite alcoholic beverages. There is some contention here. Alcohols like beer are considered a type of carbohydrate and can easily upset your daily carbohydrate macros. Still, these exist low-carb varieties of beer that would not upset daily carbs by much. Drinking alcohol on a permissive keto diet is certainly possible. Things like red wine are also low in carbs and pose many health benefits.

The main concern with alcohol on keto is binge drinking, and drinking high carbohydrate alcohol. Plus, many alcohol varieties like beer are not considered a whole food. As such, they do not make part of a strict, whole foods based keto diet. Use at your own discretion.

CHAPTER 3:

Benefits of a Ketogenic Diet

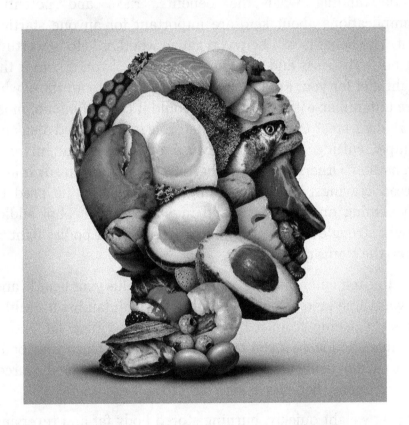

At first glance, the keto diet may not seem radically different from a standard diet. After all, people usually eat lots of meat, chicken, fish, dairy and vegetables on a regular basis. The main difference is of course, high carbohydrate foods like bread. The other difference is the allowance of processed foods, which should not be eaten on keto. By simply taking these two elements out of the diet, maintaining adequate protein consumption and ramping up the healthy fats, keto unlocks a number of benefits that are inaccessible with a standard diets. These benefits go far and wide from a health perspective. They do not simply stop at weight loss.

Understanding what the benefits, risks and potential complications about keto are important for anyone starting out. The benefits will help you gauge whether keto is worth it or not. The risks and complications will tell you if keto is the right diet for you. Keto is easy to underestimate for those who are unfamiliar with it. How hard could it be to eliminate most carbohydrates? Carbs do have their role in a balanced diet, and simply cutting them out because of keto is not an easy transition. Others will have a hard time coping with sugar and bread cravings. These are things that the body is used to consuming on daily basis and much like an alcohol addict might struggle from withdrawal, so too will our bodies fight to keep the status quo.

But this tendency must be resisted if you value your health, and if you value keto as a viable option for maintaining a healthy lifestyle. Going from a high carb diet to a high fat one is completely doable if you take the right steps. Once your body gets used to using fat both as a fuel and a primary food source, the secondary benefits of keto start to shine.

Losing weight quickly, burning stored body fat and reversing the damage from high sugar diets are the most commonly cited benefits of keto. These are the "poster boys" for the diet. But other benefits that may appear obscure to some also exist. For example, diets high in processed foods will tend to be high in sodium and sugar. Eating keto without the processed foods will help control salt intake as well as sugar.

Overall, keto is a healthy option for the majority of people out there. Some consider the carbohydrate restriction as an "extreme" diet and as a consequence keto has received the reputation of being a difficult, or even dangerous diet. There is the attitude that only health conscious nuts and people who have a neurotic personality willingly undergo keto. Still, others will stumble on the diet reading articles on the Internet. And as anyone who spends even a little bit on time online knows, not everything you read on the internet is truthful. Keto has joined other similar diets in being branded as "fringe" or wonky in nature.

There is such a deep rooted human element with eating carbohydrates that the idea of going cold turkey is perceived as crazy. And yet those same people are willing to eat processed breakfast cereals, potato chips and white flour breads. Bread and grain in particular have been considered a staple food for many peoples throughout history. Processed foods and refined carbohydrates on the other hand, are relatively new inventions in the human diet. And there is nothing intrinsically natural or human in eating them. This is perhaps where the keto diet really shines. It may be true that carbohydrates have their role in human nutrition, but it is also true that refined carbs and sugars cause weight gain and other types of harm in the long run.

Given that most people's diets are already high in refined carbs and sugars, keto is just a valid option as any. It may even be easier—at least for some—to eat a healthy, balanced diet while on keto than to do the same with a standard diet. For example, the dieter on keto knows that bread is off limits. They will not inadvertently eat a refined carb because they know it's off the table. The dieter who is not on keto must take the extra step of finding unrefined flour products, or low-carbohydrate alternatives if they wish to eat just as healthily.

Keto also isn't dangerous if done in properly. In contrast a diet high in refined sugars *is* dangerous, even if not immediately obvious. Given its high beneficiary profile, keto is well worth the perceived risk. Low-carb diets are no more harmful than standard diets are. There is no such thing as a nutrient deficiency between those who are in ketosis year round and those who prefer their carbohydrates. The only real difference is between fuel sources. We all know glucose as a fuel. We all know that too much glucose leads to diabetes. But not many of us appreciate the benefits of fat as a fuel.

Accelerated Fat Loss

Fat, or adipose tissue stored either under the skin or in organ fat is simply sugar in stealth mode. In terms of evolution, it is a useful survival mechanism. Any organism that stores excess caloric energy as fat can gorge on food when it is plentiful and still keep the rest. Otherwise that same precious food would be taken apart by scavengers and other animals competing for resources. Then when food is scarce, their bodies can slowly melt that fat back into glucose and keep their bodies going long enough to find the next big bounty.

It is possible that early humans lived in the same manner for thousands of years. Eating in times of feast and surviving in times of hunger. But adipose tissue storage gives us little advantage in the modern world. Instead it poses a disadvantage—fat tissue increases the risk of cardiovascular disease and obesity. Food scarcity simply doesn't exist in the modern world. All of us expect to eat at least three major meals a day, with snacks in between and maybe even dessert. All of this food is relatively cheap. And if cost isn't an issue, it is still highly available. Nobody in a developed country is going to starve because food isn't accessible.

A standard diet gives us a steady stream of glucose—and for the average person, a steady stream of stored fat. This is in the form of belly fat, love handles, flabby underarms, enlarged breasts in men, saggy butts, and so on. Everyone can universally identify fat on the body. This steady stream of caloric energy is almost never upset. We may skip meals inadvertently or go for a few hours without eating, but eventually we get hungry, we get irritable and then we need something to eat. This is because food is there and available. A store is always around the corner and most people live within a few miles of a fast food joint.

The consequence is that fat never gets melted down to glucose because our bodies are always full of it. Burning fat on a standard diet is notoriously difficult. Here nobody seems to have the right answers. Eat less and move more, eat more but lift weights to increase metabolism, perform lots of cardio, sweat the fat out. These are all commonly forms of advice or perceived advice that people trying to lose weight are given.

Ever so often, someone will say "eat less bread", and this will resonate for a little while but quickly be forgotten within the next meal. It isn't just bread that makes you fat, but a whole host of refined carbohydrates that run rampant in our modern pantries, grocery stores and restaurants.

When you limit carbs and go into ketosis, fat is already being burned without being converted into glucose. The keto diet requires some 65% of calories or more to be derived from fats because it will be the new form of glucose that your bode uses. You may recognize that this is also a steady stream of caloric energy, but remember that dietary fat isn't the same as adipose tissue. Eating health sources of fat does not immediately get converted into body fat in turn. They are first broken down into fatty acids, which can then be converted into various energy sources like ketones before finally being converted into adipose tissue if there are leftovers.

Fat in general is a much more efficient fuel source for the body. Glucose absorption is governed by the interplay of various hormones, including insulin and its counterpart glucagon. In individuals with higher levels of insulin insensitivity, glucose uptake becomes strained. On the other hand, there is no such hormonal response with the absorption of fat, and fat doesn't enter the bloodstream all at once like with glucose. Instead, fat is absorbed periodically, either getting converted into sugars or ketone bodies for ketosis.

The metabolic pathways for using fat as a primary fuel compete with the metabolic pathways for using carbohydrates. This means that the more your body becomes used to using fat for energy to better it will utilize it. Glucose is primarily influenced by insulin—if insulin prohibits the uptake of glucose either because the cells are full or because of insulin insensitivity, then the glucose gets converted into fat. Insulin must effectively be "turned off" for the body to metabolize dietary fat and prevent the long term storage of glucose.

The end result is that less glucose gets turned into adipose tissue, meanwhile ketosis is burning away at available fat stores. Here your metabolism directly influences how stored fat is used. It doesn't have to enter the complex metabolic pathway that turns adipose tissue into glucose. It doesn't have to check for insulin levels that dictate how much of that same glucose should be used as energy and how much should be stored.

Improved Energy Athletic Performance

When your body burns fat instead of glucose, something magical happens in terms of exercise. Normally, the body will turn towards glucose to fuel workout sessions. This is why some athletes will eat a carby meal hours before they plan to exercise. It provides them with adequate energy to see through a difficult routine. But what sometimes happens is that this energy tapers off in the middle of the workout, bringing performance to a crawl. Almost nobody is a stranger to this effect in the gym. Out of nowhere it seems like you are desperately tired, and you can't push yourself to finish the workout. Your glucose stores have been depleted, and your body needs more to go on. In that scenario we are more likely to end the workout, go home and regroup.

To make up for its dependency on glucose our body can store some of it in the form of glycogen. It is an intermediary between pure close and adipose tissue, usually stored in the liver and muscle cells. Glycogen doesn't get used unless the body requires immediate energy expenditure, like when running after prey in the wild. In the gym, glycogen is most likely to be used up when lifting weights or doing intense cardio sessions. And when all the glycogen is inevitably used up, our bodies feel like they can no longer go on.

In contrast, the process of ketosis provides ample energy that isn't likely to run out like glycogen. Instead of stopping in the middle of the workout you might feel fine throughout. You won't experience any unanticipated drops in blood sugar, which can ruin athletic performance.

This further translates to activities outside of the gym. We are all too familiar with the mid-afternoon crash that happens in the hours between lunch and dinner. Even if we aren't hungry, we start to feel tired and taking a nap in the middle of the office suddenly feels like a good idea. Blood sugar is usually to blame. Even if your body doesn't signal that it is running on empty, it could still be the case that blood sugar is dropping and that you are experience a mild instance of hypoglycemia. The symptoms are feeling tired, irritable or angry with decreased brain function and alertness. Since glucose supply has fallen, your body is compensating by shutting off non-vital activity like mood regulation.

Most will simply reach for another coffee to get over the slump. Others will turn to a sugary or salty snack that is high in refined carbs. It gets them through the rest of the work day until dinner comes around, but the meal can be more detrimental than that. Instead of training your body to eat nutritious, filling food such behavior encourages fluctuations in blood sugar. A small, but energetically dense meal translates to instantaneous energy at the cost of stability. You will continue to experience the same crash unless those eating habits are changed.

Since blood sugar fluctuation doesn't really affect you while on ketosis, the mid-afternoon slump is rare. You can stay productive for eight hours or more during the day and still have more left for doing things outside of work. And you won't feel like dying half way between dinner.

Increased Focus and Cognitive Ability

Your brain on fat is like being a completely different you. Mental alertness on the ketogenic diet is like taking a hit of caffeine every hour of the day, and it has little to do with the bulletproof coffee. It is no wonder that the same diet used to treat various neurological disorders like epilepsy can also be used to enhance mental capabilities. It a booster of overall brain health. And while it probably won't make you a genius or raise IQ by a few points, you can still benefit from a clearly thinking brain.

Epilepsy is usually attributed to an overactive brain, or certain regions of the brain that become overexcited for no reason. There seems to be some connection between the over excitation and standard diets which may include refined carbs and sugar. Those who go on keto report feeling more mellow overall, with reduced rates of anxiety and fastidiousness.

Memory improves, regardless of age. Others have reported treating their migraines and cluster headaches by going on low-carb diets such as keto. In addition, mental clarity is at an all time high, driving a better ability to focus for longer periods of time.

Sugar Detoxification

Let's get something clear. Sugar in large amounts is toxic to our bodies. Molecularly speaking, every carbohydrate is a type of sugar and not just the sweet tasting stuff we normally associate with sugar. When no precaution is taken to limit refined carbs or sugar in the diet, disastrous things can happen to your health. Many already recognize this as increased fat storage, but fewer consider the ramifications of type 2 diabetes and obesity. Everyone is scared silly about their cholesterol levels and eating greasy food, but nobody talks about the possible dangers of the humble carbohydrate. Among type 2 diabetics, more of them will die of heart related complications than the other commonly cited complications like kidney failure. High sugar diets raise the risk of cardiovascular disease in diabetics because high concentrations of sugar in the arteries can create blockages in the form of calcified blood vessels. Diabetes fear heart attack and stroke more than they do dialysis.

Conditions like fatty liver disease are accelerated by the presence of adipose tissue within the organ walls. In the liver these fat cells come from excess sugar that they fail to convert into energy. First sugar will get stored as glycogen in the liver, former a quick-melting reserve of energy for when we go a few hours without eating. But once glycogen stores as at their maximum capacity, the liver has no choice but to turn the glucose into fat. A simple search online for healthy liver vs fatty liver will give you all the information that you need to know. The only way that this organ borne fat can be reduced is through diet. No matter of exercise will burn visceral fat in a noticeable way.

Over time, a keto diet will slowly but surely start to rid the liver of excess sugar. For some this will be a painful process as their bodies go into a state of sugar withdrawal. But in the end their livers will thank them for it. And while the liver is normally associated with detoxification of alcohol, it has little mechanisms for detoxing itself from pent up sugar.

Decreased Cardiovascular Risk

Diets high in carbohydrates directly raise bad cholesterol by forming excess triglycerides when excess glucose can't be absorbed. The effect is even worse in individuals with insulin insensitivity problems, wherein glucose has a harder time being metabolized into energy. Going on a keto diet lowers this production of triglycerides due to an influx in carbs.

What's more, keto acts as an anti-inflammatory diet. Using whole foods that are high in antioxidants helps keep long term inflammation down. Inflammation is just as risky to cardiovascular disease as is cholesterol or triglycerides build up.

A Cure For Aging

Finally, keto in conjunction with intermittent fasting, (which will be covered later in this book) may help prevent aging. Observational studies both in animal models and humans have found a correlation between calorie restriction and longevity. Some of the oldest people on earth always enjoy a sparse diet, and scientist weren't really sure why. From an non-scientific standpoint it sort of does make sense that eating a little bit will help you live for longer. Your body undergoes less metabolic and digestive stress from eating. A modern equivalent would be a car that is driven often, and with a heavy foot. Frequent hard brakes and acceleration spikes correlate with frequent blood sugar and insulin spikes. Over time a heavy foot will damage the engine and transmission of a car so that its operational life is lower than that of a car driven with more care.

Hints as to why a low calorie diet makes people live for longer could be found in the ketone body β-hydroxybutyrate, which is present during times of starvation. The same ketone body is also present during prolonged fasts, long exercise sessions, and of course during ketosis. B-hydroxybutyrate can further block certain enzyme histone deacetylases, (HDC's) which are responsible for causing genetic damage in the long term. It could be that low calorie diets, fasting and ketogenic diets all have similar properties which are spurred by the ketone body B-hydroxybutyrate.

CHAPTER 4:

Risks and Complications, Who Should and Shouldn't be on Keto

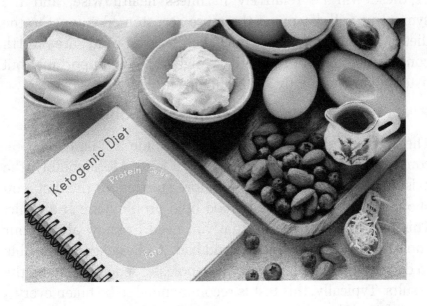

Switching to keto is an overall healthy way of jump starting a new diet, but it may not be for everyone. As with any weight loss routine, there are risks and potential health considerations that the dieter needs to be aware of. These considerations are in no way aimed to scare off would be dieters or to "weed out" less dedicated individuals. Instead they are presented to help you make informed decisions with your diet and with your health. Weight loss isn't something you can address with a band-aid approach. If there are existing issues with your health, simply using your diet as a cure all may cause leaks somewhere else.

There is some truth to the keto critics who say that it is an extreme diet. Most of us are accustomed to diets that are high in carbohydrates. And regardless if carbs are quintessential to human nutrition or not, getting off the carbohydrate train will come at a cost. The previous chapter covered some of the benefits of the diet, this chapter will cover some of the negative things you may come to expect when making the switch. Many of these will be relatively harmless health wise, and the symptoms will disappear the more accustomed you get to the diet. Other issues are may be serious, and are worth considering for your health. Weight loss is important, but listening to one's body and wellbeing always comes first.

Risks Involving Preexisting Medical Conditions

The biggest threat to your health will come from any medical condition that doesn't play nice with keto. Most notably, the existence of high cholesterol. Before starting on the diet, you should definitely get a full blood lipid profile done at a clinic. This test will give you all that you need to know about your cholesterol levels, both good and bad. A physician will be able to diagnose you with high or low cholesterol depending on the results. Typically, this test is recommended to be taken every 5 years for adults with otherwise good health.

Your blood lipid profile will tell you how much HDL and LDL is in your blood stream. People often confuse these two indicators to mean cholesterol in blood. In fact, neither HDL or LDL are types of cholesterol. See, fat is very water phobic and could never travel through the bloodstream on its own. Instead, it hitches a ride on the backs of lipoproteins, of which there is a high-density and low-density variety. Low-density lipoproteins are called "bad cholesterol" because they are smaller compared to HDL and have the possibility of getting stuck in the arteries. LDL carries cholesterol to the cells so that they can produce hormones and do all sorts of stuff. HDL ferries cholesterol through the blood and into the liver, where it will either be recycled or ferried back into the intestines to get turned into waste. Furthermore, because of their physical size, HDL's can help move LDL along and get them unstuck. This is why getting a full blood lipid profile is important. You could have high cholesterol, but still have a healthy ratio of HDL to LDL. Our bodies can produce up to 75% of cholesterol needs on their own. The rest we get comes from the food we eat.

Sine a keto diet is already high in things like animal proteins and fats, raising cholesterol levels is a real concern for many. In particular, raising LDL and its evil twin, VLDL. Also called very low-density lipoproteins, VLDL's are even smaller than regular LDL and more likely to get stuck in between arterial walls. VLDL's carry triglycerides (fat) rather than cholesterol. Given that increased levels of cholesterol are often reported with the keto diet, someone with a worrisome blood lipid profile may wish to consult a doctor before going on the diet.

Cholesterol itself doesn't effect cardiovascular risk because our bodies normally know how to regulate it. What causes problems, though, are LDL's and VLDL's. They are what clog arteries, not necessarily the cholesterol that they transport. A keto diet, despite raising overall cholesterol levels, can bring down VLDL levels and enlarge the size of the LDL and VLDL particles. This is because a diet high in carbohydrates will produce excess glucose. When cells don't need anymore energy, the glucose molecules first get converted into triglycerides, which then get stored as adipose tissue. Going low-carb limits glucose intake, and less triglycerides enter the bloodstream in this way. Diets high in carbohydrates not only increase triglycerides, but they also decrease particle size for LDL, meanwhile increasing the number of individual particles.

There is a case for going on keto to reduce the overall risk of cardiovascular disease, as strange as it sounds. It deals with closely monitoring cholesterol levels and eating healthy fats. Cholesterol may go up, but triglycerides and particle size will go down. And it really is important to take blood lipid profiles more often while on keto, just to make sure everything is in check. If constantly checking for blood lipids and other health indicators sounds like too daunting a task, then maybe keto isn't for you.

Diabetes

The other major health risk is for those who are currently suffering from either type 1 or type 2 diabetes. With the high blood sugar levels of diabetes and the necessary medication to bring it down, diabetes sufferers may subject themselves to dangerous instances of hypoglycemia. These individuals should definitely consult a doctor before making any major dietary changes. Since keto limits carbs, the insulin medications taken by both type 1 and type 2 diabetics may lower glucose too much.

Secondly, diabetics are at an increased risk of developing ketoacidosis, a potentially life threatening version of ketosis. In ketoacidosis, ketone bodies such as β-hydroxybutyrate and acetoacetic acid flood the bloodstream in large amounts, causing a toxicity in the body. The condition is characterized by dehydration and an inability to get glucose to cells that need them. It is prone to affect sufferers of type 1 diabetes more than type 2 because of their inability to create insulin on their own. It is also possible to develop ketoacidosis by consuming large amounts of alcohol, which will cause dehydration. Other causes include fat being broken down too quickly, or the liver creating large amounts of glucose at once, such that cells can't absorb them all.

Symptoms of ketoacidosis involve feeling faint, quickened breathing, loss of alertness, nausea and vomiting, headaches, muscle soreness and frequent urination in particular. If diagnosed early and treated promptly, ketoacidosis is highly treatable. But if the symptoms are ignored, complications may include kidney failure, heart attack and stroke.

Despite the potential risks, type 2 diabetics have much to benefit from a keto diet. A possible way that type 2 diabetes occurs is because the diet is high in carbs and sugars in the first place . Going on keto, glucose levels drop on their own because blood sugar spikes virtually stop, and the related insulin response also goes down. Over time, a type 2 diabetic may not even need to take insulin regularly to control their blood sugar levels because the keto diet is taking care of it for them. This usually doesn't mean that keto can cure the disease—only help manage it. As soon as the diabetic returns to eating their carbohydrate rich foods, chronic hyperglycemia returns.

Still, the keto lifestyle may be a healthy alternative to standard diabetes medication. Low-carb diets have been used to treat diabetes for a long time, and keto is no different. The diabetic wishing to try keto should know how to regularly check their blood sugar levels, blood lipid profile, and the presence of ketone bodies. The last bit is important, because ketoacidosis can be detected early on if ketone bodies rise beyond a certain level.

Various Other Conditions

It still worth getting your doctors approval if you suffer from different diseases and or conditions. The keto diet may not be suited for young children or adolescents (unless those individuals are obese or substantially overweight). The elderly and those over the age of 55 may also want to check in with their primary care physicians before attempting the diet.

Anyone who suffers from liver conditions, pancreas conditions or problems with their kidneys should also have caution. Other conditions that are sensitive to changes in nutrition should also be included. Cancer patients and suffers from other chronic diseases will need to talk with their doctors as well before starting keto. All of these individuals are at an increased risk of developing the symptoms listed below. If at any point these symptoms become severe, it is time to stop the diet and or seek immediate medical advice.

Effects of a Keto Diet

Making the transition to low carb is never easy. Just like an alcoholic faces withdrawal symptoms if they stop taking it, so too will anyone trying to get off their carbohydrate or sugar fixations. Thankfully, the symptoms of carbohydrate withdrawal are relatively tame compared to those associated with alcohol. But they are difficult enough to get through that many consider quitting the diet before experiencing ketosis. Know that whatever symptoms you do feel are not characteristic of the diet itself, but that they are due to your body making the switch to fat burning. Immediately after eating your last non-ketogenic meal you will feel the usual symptoms of falling blood sugar. You will feel things like being tired or irritable because you haven't eaten in a while. You may also experience mild headaches or brain fog. Overall, you will feel sluggish like if your energy levels are dropping. This is to be expected, because normally we eat food to get a burst of energy when we need it. Besides taking a nap, getting more calories in is the only way feel normal again. Except with keto you won't be consuming carbs—and your body will hate you for it. At least, for the first couple of days on the diet.

How long the transition period will vary between people, and will especially depend on how much refined carbs and sugar they get on their normal diet. It could last anywhere from a few days to a week, but typically no more than three days. What people feel during this time will also vary in severity. Some experience strong symptoms that scare them off from the diet. Others only have mild ones, and these are usually forgotten. If your body has a negative reaction to getting off carbohydrates then relax—it is just going through a sugar detoxification process. Your liver is getting freed from the sugar stores it has hoarded up fro years. But if negative symptoms persist or get noticeably worse during the first few days, it could be a sign that the diet simply isn't for you. Listen to your body and pay attention to what it tells you. The combination of symptoms experienced during the first few days are known colloquially as the keto flu. And this name has persisted, despite the fact that many of the symptoms aren't flu like at all. A lucky few won't experience negative symptoms at all, or else feel just a tiny bit of what others do. But usually they can range from feelings of dizzyness and weakness, tiredness and general lethargy. More worrying symptoms include headaches, changes in mood, difficulty sleeping and trouble staying alert. Severe symptoms may include diarrhea, vomiting, stomach pains and muscle soreness.

If either diarrhea or vomiting present themselves frequently or if they increase in intensity, the diet should be put on hold until normal conditions return. The presence of either symptom may be a serious medical issue. One can quickly lose fluids through diarrhea and vomiting which could lead to an emergency.

What Can You do to Make the Transition Easier

Some of the symptoms of keto flu may have an underlying cause that you can treat. Not getting enough water, for example, can exacerbate things like diarrhea and vomiting. As you make the transition, make sure you are keeping your fluids up. To be on the safe side, drink a little bit more than you would normally do. Always strive to get plenty of rest, even if insomnia occurs. Getting adequate sleep will help keep your energy levels stable throughout the day.

Another possible underlying cause is an electrolyte imbalance from the switch in diet. Electrolytes are the minerals we normally get from our diets. The main ones are sodium, potassium, magnesium and calcium. Fruits are a good source for electrolytes but unfortunately you won't be eating too much of them with keto. At least not without doing some serious carbohydrate counting. Drinking more water and especially mineral water will help keep electrolytes normal. Avoid any popular sugary sports drink.

For the time being, avoid any strenuous exercise that may exacerbate these symptoms. Wait until the ketosis period kicks in, then you can exercise until near exhaustion without fear of inducing a serious hypoglycemia attack.

Finally, a little will power never hurt anyone. Someone who has enjoyed a diet high in refined carbs and sugar for most of their life should know what they are getting into. It is these people who typically have the worst time making the transition. And just like the alcoholic seeking rehabilitation, the withdrawal is often brutal. You will get sugar cravings all throughout the process. Your best bet is to stick to your will, keep yourself busy and power through the keto flu.

Food Allergies

Lastly, as with any diet, compatibility will be dictated by how well your body reacts to certain foods. Keto is a good option for those with gluten intolerances, as you won't be eating any bread. Other food allergies, like lactose intolerance, are more tricky with the keto diet. Note that dairy products are commonly used in keto recipes. Some people may have difficulty eating pork or beef. These can be supplanted by using chicken and fish, but that may not be sustainable for some people. Make sure you know which foods you can eat, and which of those are allowed on keto. A good match will be no dairy intolerance, and the ability to eat all types of meat.

Others can't eat certain foods because of religious purposes. Muslims aren't allowed to eat pork, for example and some cultures prohibit the consumption of beef. Environmentally conscious and animal friendly dieters may bawk at the idea of eating meat or mass produced fish. This presents a problem for the vegan or vegetarian keto dieter because getting enough fat, protein and electrolytes is difficult on a low-carb vegan or vegetarian diet. Such dieting configurations have been pulled off in the past, though. And there is a plethora of online vegan keto resources available.

Even when such intolerances are present, it only takes a little creativity to alter the diet to your liking. A food intolerance doesn't bar you from keto outright, but it may make things a little more difficult.

CHAPTER 5:

Keto Diet for Weight Loss

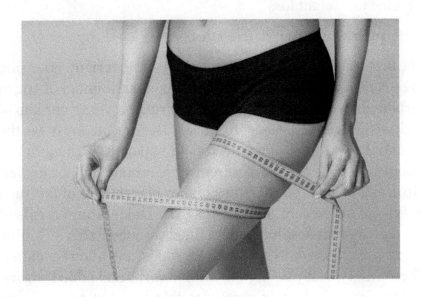

L osing weight with keto is easy by virtue of the low carb, high fat diet. Diet is the most important factor of weight loss, all other things being equal. This means that no matter of exercise will amount to results compared to what you eat. Following a strict keto diet already does most of the guesswork for you. You won't have to second guess which foods are good for you and which aren't. You are limiting carbohydrates, thereby limiting glucose intake. At the same time, you are getting most of your calories from healthy fats, helping drive those metabolic pathways behind ketosis.

Weight loss is a simple function of diet, exercise, and meal timing. All three compliment each other to various degrees, and all three will be covered throughout this book. Diet is an obvious factor, because it derives how many calories we receive from food, and what macro nutrient composition that food is made from. Then there's exercise, the much dreaded but necessary form of deliberate calorie use. Lastly, there is meal timing, which is usually ignored by dieting advice but still packs a punch for weight loss.

Getting in Tune with the Diet

The first step towards weight loss is getting diet right. For a diet to be considered "ketogenic" it must have a minimum of 50g of carbohydrates, adequate protein (typically 1.5 – 2g per kilo of bodyweight) and the rest from fat. Dietary fat must be the essential part of the diet, and should make up the majority of calories. Usually the fat requirement is around 65% or higher. More astute keto followers use higher percentages of fat, such as 80 and 90 percent. Beyond that, the major requirements of the diet are that absolutely no refined carbohydrates including sugar are allowed. No processed foods are allowed either. These will typically be high in refined carbs and added sugars, so the first rule largely precludes this one, but many forget about it.

The first question people ask is how in the world are they supposed to get upwards to 70% or more of their daily calories from fat. For the uninitiated, it seems like a daunting task. But since fat is so high in calories to begin with, you will be amazed at how quickly you can ramp them up.

Next they ask about carbs. What does a 50g or lower in carbohydrates look like? Realistically, a healthy keto diet will contain around 25g to 50g of carbs, but they shouldn't come from things like grains. Fruits are allowed, but are frowned upon because of high carbohydrate contents. These 50g carbs you are allowed should be put towards calculating the net carbohydrates of vegetables, which are simply the carbohydrate content minus fiber. So if one cup of spinach has 6g of carbs but 2g fiber, the net carbohydrates are 4g. This is the number you count towards the either 25g or 50g requirement.

Proteins come in all shapes and sizes, but are generally used to refer to meat. Other types of protein, like legumes are also high in carbohydrates, and will quickly surpass the 50g baseline for many foods. Be careful that meat isn't prepared in such a way that will raise the overall carbohydrate content. Breaded chicken is a big offender. Fried varieties will have a low carbohydrate count, but may still add up if you are not careful.

No Processed Foods, refined carbs or sugar

Shopping for keto is easy, keeping in mind the restrictions mentioned above. No refined carbs, no sugar, no processed foods. The aim with the diet is to use whole ingredients wherever possible. Sometimes this may be difficult, or there may be a specialty food that is ketogenic but is still processed. Your mileage may vary when choosing these foods. There is one school of keto that says that the stricter the diet the better. There is another that says the easier to follow the diet is, then the better for the individual. If various food products and recipes out there are designed to make keto more palatable, then it may be worth using them in your diet. But be warned that some of these recipes and products are either processed goods or are using them in some matter.

A processed good—as the name implies—is anything that has been "processed" by a manufacturer. And they certainly don't grow on trees. These products will usually come packaged in someway, but not all packaged items are processed, which can make things tricky. For example, if you go to a local grocer or farmer's market they might sell you homemade jam in little jars. They are certainly packaged food, but are all natural. While they may be mechanically processed or pressed in such a way to make the jam, they have zero added chemicals or sugars. In cases like this, identifying a processed good comes down to judgment and or the history of the product life cycle. A local seller will always be able to tell you where the food came from, what was done to it and how long ago. If you try doing that at a supermarket you will have no such luck.

Inevitably this means ransacking your current fridge or pantry to get rid of various snacks, breakfast cereals, cookies, and so on. People with existing sugar or carbohydrate addictions will have the hardest time making the transition. But once they are a few months into the diet, their sugar cravings will wane. Sugar or sugar derived products can no longer be used for cooking, baking, or preparing food in any way. Sugary drinks are also out of the question. People on keto nominally drink water, mineral water, water infusions, tea, and coffee. Anything else is pushing the envelope.

The line of what is good to eat on keto also gets blurred when eating prepared meals or eating out. Chicken is nominally a very good keto food as long as it is prepared in a keto friendly way. When you buy a rotisserie chicken at the grocery store though, you have little knowledge of how the chicken was prepared. Sometimes there will be a label telling you what kind of seasoning was used, or if there are any preservatives in the marinade. Other times you won't get this information. The rotisserie chicken may still come in a plastic container of some sort—but it doesn't mean it is processed. Eating at a restaurant is a similar conundrum. The best way to maintain a strict keto diet is to prepare all your meals, but sometimes life gets in the way. There exists a variety of keto friendly delivery services and food prep services that you may wish to use.

A restaurant isn't always compelled to tell you the ingredients beforehand. Sometimes you can tell what a certain dish entails. A sweet and sour pork dish is probably not going to be keto. Your best bet is to talk with the waiter about what the dish contains. And if they can't give you a straight answer, it is best to err on the side of caution.

Eating the right things while on keto is critical for weight loss. Any weakness in the diet will inevitably show up as weakness in weight loss results. This is because processed foods, refined carbs and sugar all encourage fat storage. Even eating at your caloric requirements with some of these foods is a bad idea— the insulin insensitivity factor still plays a role. The standard keto diet allows a maximum of 50g of carbohydrates, none of which should be of the refined variety. It is even possible to drop this requirement to 0g of carbs, or to keep it as low as possible. The lower this number, the easier it will be to stay in ketosis.

What If I Have a Sweet Tooth?

Keto friendly snacks do exist, but implementing them into your diet is never straight forward. The issue comes with sugar, and the processed nature of artificial sweeteners. People on keto might elect to make an oily, fat based snack called a "fat bomb". They are typically high in coconut oil, or some other palatable fat source. For taste, such ingredients as cocoa powder, vanilla extract and artificial sweeteners are often added. These additives are controversial from a keto perspective—a strict keto diet shouldn't allow them, but they are still used by people who say that they are on the diet. Sugar gives a food its sweet taste, period. But these additives do not contain sugar as per the label. Vanilla extracts are typically made with an ethanol base, which is no different from adding a dash of rum to your morning coffee. All natural vanilla extracts exist, and they are advertised as having "zero sugar". If that is true, where does the sweet taste come from?

Fruit is naturally sweet, by virtue of the sugar called fructose. So even if it is all natural, it isn't necessarily "sugar free". Be suspicious of any sweet tasting product that is labeled as sugar free. It may indicate that there is no sucrose (regular table sugar, one glucose and one fructose molecule) present in the food. But it may use some alternative sweetener. And the world of artificial sweeteners is a wacky world of chemical concoctions. Here hard-line keto followers are more likely to defend their sugar habits by saying that artificial sweeteners are fine. And yet, artificial sweeteners are a processed good. The quest for sweet tasting food is that powerful.

Whether you use artificial sweeteners like sucralose or erythritol is up to you. Some artificial sweeteners found in diet sodas have been associated with increased cardiovascular risk. They don't raise glucose levels outright, but they may increase insulin insensitivity, especially if consumed regularly. Ask yourself this: if artificial sweeteners are so harmless, then why do people feel guilty about drinking zero calorie sodas that are still loaded with them? Why do we look down upon people who are "dieting" but still drink one or two of these sodas a day? Because we know, by some instinctual means, that these products are not healthy. No doctor will recommend you to drink these products on a regular basis. They are already familiar with the scientific literature that says they are harmful. Even natural sweeteners may have some chemical processing added to them before entering the final product.

For some this may feel like a witch hunt against all that is sweet. The goal of any keto diet should be to harness a healthier lifestyle. And sugar is often part of an unhealthy lifestyle, especially once it becomes an addiction. Eating the occasional keto snack probably isn't that bad for you, even if it uses some artificial sweetener. But it has to remain an "occasional snack", not something you indulge in all the time. There is no cheating with keto. You are either on keto, or you are not.

The other major factor to keep in mind is ease of use. If using certain ingredients, whether processed or not makes following a standard keto diet easier, then by all means use them. But use them with caution. The trade-off works if you stay off refined carbs and follow a lower than 50g daily carb requirement. Whatever processed goods or artificial sweeteners you use will pale in comparison.

In recent years keto has become big business. This means a mass of new products have hit mainstream grocery shelves like Wal-Mart, Target and Costco in the United States. It speaks volumes about the newfound popularity of the diet, but most of these products have their own drawbacks. Making your own keto "bars" will always be healthier than buying some iof the processed ones you can get at the store. Keto works best when you use all whole ingredients, and many of these products have artificial sweeteners and other additives thrown into the mix. One must question if these products are even keto, or if they are simply trying to pander to a new audience of quasi health conscious consumers. If people see the label "keto" they will automatically think it is healthy. But this is no different from the advertising machine behind "sugar free" products and "healthy" snacks that hit the market during the past few decades.

Keto does not belong in a box, but many people will say that it does. The original philosophy of keto diets was that they required healthy ingredients, and a low carbohydrate profile. The stuff you buy at the store may have low-carbs, but it doesn't mean it is good for you. Keto, being an emerging trend, is attracting tons of capital expenditure from companies seeking to make an easy buck. Healthy food is a commodity they wish to sell you, already prepackaged and prepared for your liking. But you are paying from something that isn't necessary. Indulging in the occasional commercial keto bars, protein powders, fat bombs and other processed concoctions is fine, so long as they are used for supplementation. These products are not replacements for the real thing, and should not be relied on for the long term.

Keto at the Grocery Store

When you go about setting up your ketogenic pantry, you will have to navigate the endless isles of grocery store junk. This is often easier said that done, especially because many do not know which foods are adequate for keto and which ones are not. A good start is removing refined carbs, processed foods and sugars. Next, pick food that is whole and nutritious. Avoid anything that has "empy calories". Anything that you put in your mouth should provide you with a net benefit, not a guilty pleasure.

Whole foods are easy to spot because they seem like something you could easily find in nature or in an agricultural setting. They may still come packaged in plastic, but that doesn't mean they are processed. Look for leafy greens, healthy fat sources (more on that in a bit), quality meats and low-carb alternatives for food that you love. Keto doesn't have to be overly expensive, or any more expensive than your regular meal. Yes, carby and processed food is often cheaper than the whole food variety, but costs taper off when you find cheap alternatives. Nobody says you have to eat prime rib for dinner everyday to do keto. Nobody says you must use chicken breast or top salmon fillet for every recipe. Cheaper cuts of meat, such as chicken thighs, ground beef and chuck roast are trivial to find. In many cases, they provide about the same nutritional value than their more expensive counterparts.

Remember that proteins aren't the focus of the diet. The standard keto diet requires that you receive adequate protein for your weight, and no more. Those who wish to use a modified, high-protein keto diet can do so at their own discretion. Higher protein requirements will mean they have to either supplement the difference or to eat more meat. This will invariably result in a higher grocery bill than regular keto.

Fats are relatively cheap compared to animal protein because you get more metabolic bang for your buck. Dairy products like cheeses and creams may be used to cover both protein and fat requirements at once. If you are lactose intolerant though, this route may not be available to you and you will have to look for alternative ways to getting the most out of your shopping experience.

In the Meat Aisle

A standard keto meal is usually based around a meat. The animal proteins found in beef, poultry, pork and fish are slow digesting and keep you psychologically fuller for longer. Most of the meat you find at the butcher shop or meat aisle is good to eat on keto. Yes, they come wrapped in plastic, but aren't typically a processed food. More stringent dieters may decide to use organic and grass fed varieties but these will be more expensive. Don't worry so much about the fat content of the various cuts. Fatty beef is allowed, so is chicken with the skin still intact. In fact, these are often encouraged because they help you reach daily fat requirements quickly. Fatty cuts will of course, raise cholesterol.

Beef and red meat is also notorious for raising cholesterol levels, but this shouldn't be a problem for most people. After all, people on keto have a better HDL to LDL ratio, with lesser risk of cardiovascular disease than people with high carbohydrate diets. Most of the American population is lacking in good HDL numbers, which can be raised by going on keto. There are many different cuts of beef, lamb and pork that you may wish to use. Buy the cheapest ones, if money is an issue. All of them are more or less the same for the purposes of the diet. Buy cuts with bones included if you wish to make bone broths, stocks, or stews for your diet.

Avoid buying cured meat, unless you know for a fact they are keto friendly. Sausages, pepperoni, deli meats and even bacon come in processed varieties. Bacon and sausage show up time and time again in keto recipes, so it is important that you know the right stuff to buy. Cured meats including hot dogs and bacon contain sulfites which are a possible carcinogen. These foods can be enjoyed from time to time, but do so at your own risk. Bacon is high in sodium and nitrates, as are the other cured meats. For keto this may be good because the sodium content will make it easier to balance your electrolytes. Or in some cases, bacon may contain sugar. It is best to read the label on your favorite brands and see which ones contain sugar and which ones don't. However, bacon isn't used in large servings, and will rarely (if ever) constitute as a main dish. Bacon is used more as a snack, as a flavor additive or a side dish. The relatively small serving sizes associated with eating bacon makes it safe to eat in moderate amounts.

Eggs, while not technically a meat, still serve the same concerns that meats do. That they are high in vitamins and minerals and protein is often overlooked because they are also high in fat in cholesterol. But eggs are relatively harmless both in the medical literate and in the keto diet. Many consider eggs to be a super food, whether they come from chickens, quail, or even ostrich. Furthermore, eggs are one of the cheapest protein sources that money can buy. You can get them wholesale at warehouse retailers like Costco. Organic and grass fed varieties are also available, but are by no means necessary for a healthy diet. There is no shortage of recipes that call for eggs in the keto diet. You can hard boil them, dice them up and enjoy them in a salad, or eat the boiled egg whole as a snack or side dish. You can eat them scrambled, deviled, sunnyside up and so on. Eggs are a versatile food, and a staple in the keto diet.

Chicken and fish provide good alternatives to red beef, either because of cholesterol concerns or because of taste. Chicken breast is used in many recipes, second only to chicken thighs. Purchase a whole chicken if you wish to make broths, soups or stews. Turkey is another type of poultry that you can use like chicken, in conjunction with duck and various other game birds. A common complaint is that chicken has a bland taste, especially in regards to chicken breast. If you have such a concern, you may season your dishes with salt and pepper and other keto friendly spices and sauces. The protein content of chicken breast and red meat is about the same, so it doesn't matter which you chose to eat. On the whole, a lean cut of chicken will contain less fat than a lean cut of red meat, but both meats have similar effects on cholesterol.

Fish and seafood are also keto favorites. They have a different taste from the other meats and may be used to change up the diet from time to time. Fish and seafood tend to be more expensive than the cheapest cuts of chicken and meat. Tilapia, trout and salmon are good options for entrées. Shrimp, while a little high in cholesterol, also make for great dinner platters and side dishes. Sushi in general is not keto friendly because it comes loaded with carbohydrates. But keto friendly varieties do exist. Shashimi is a type of plain raw sushi that is served by most sushi places. It usually comes with a side of rice though, which obviously you couldn't eat with keto. Canned fish like tuna and sardines are also used by some keto dieters but they are controversial from a whole foods approach. Still, because they are cheap and high in protein they make for great options for people in a hurry. Sometimes on the keto diet you will have to make compromises and decide for yourself if a certain food is worth eating.

Salmon is high in omega-3 fatty acids, which is a heart healthy fat. It can be eaten roasted, smoked, baked and several other ways. It is recommended to eat salmon at least twice a week. There are several species of salmon available as well as different cuts of fillets. Some vary in taste but generally they all have a similar nutritional value. Free range salmon will be more expensive than the more commonly farmed alternative, but tend to be the healthier option. Canned salmon is also available, but lacks some of the nutritional content found in the whole food kind.

When buying meat, you will want to purchase a select combination of meats and cuts. Make sure you know what your favorites are, and what go to dishes you eat every week. This will make shopping easier in the long run so that you only have to buy certain cuts. If you need to go the cheaper route, don't be afraid of purchasing meat in bulk or from the cheaper cuts. A few pounds of beef chuck roast can take you a long way, same for whole chickens which tend to be more affordable than specific cuts. In a pinch, rotisserie chicken are even cheaper than the raw whole chickens. This chicken can be enjoyed as is or you can remove the skin and pull the chicken into shreds for other dishes.

In the Produce Section

The next obvious stop on your grocery trip will be to the produce section. Here you will find an ample supply of fresh greens, fruits and non-starchy veggies. There will also be some restrictions to what you should buy. Since carbohydrates are out, starchy vegetables like potatoes are not allowed in your pantry. A single white potato may have as much as 33g of carbs, which is already in excess of the 20g carb requirement and more than half of the 50g carb requirement. Sweet potatoes may have a lesser carb content, but not by much. Avoid both of these in your shopping lists, unless you are making the occasional meal with sweet potatoes (even then, don't use too much per serving size). An even better alternative is to use butter squash, which has about 16g of carbs per cup. Some non-starchy vegetables can be used in place of starchy ones. Mushrooms, cauliflower and squash may have a similar consistency to potatoes.

For the most part, you are going to avoid picking fruits. Things like apples, bananas and pears are high in cabs (thanks fructose!). These may still be enjoyed in smaller portions on your keto diet. For example, if a whole apple contains 20 some grams of carbs, half an apple will be around 10 grams, which is doable with a 50g carbohydrate limit. But it doesn't meant that all fruits are off limits. Berries are keto favorites, and you should be sure to include these in your pantry. You can buy either the raw kind or the frozen type. Both are more or less the same thing. Berries (raspberries, blueberries, and strawberries) typically only have a few carbohydrates (3-9) per 1 cup serving. Plus they are high in antioxidants, fiber, and vitamins and minerals. Berries are pretty much a keto friendly super food. They help lower inflammation (which keto already helps lower) and may be preventative of many diseases. You can eat them as is, blend them up into a smoothie, or enjoy them as a side dish to many recipes.

Besides berries you can also try plums (6g carbs per fruit), clementines (8g) and peaches (13g). When people first hear that they are not allowed to eat fruits on keto, many are taken aback. Aren't fruits natural and safe to eat? Haven't humans been eating them for centuries? In a sense yes, but hardly in large quantities. Early hunter gathered ate fruit when it was available, which wasn't all the time. Fruit was also seen as food for the wealthy across many cultures, not something that made up the standard diet. In contrast, staple foods that were available to the greatest common denominators were universally carbohydrate rich or starchy. It isn't so much that fruit is bad, it's that the sugars found within them are not compatible with the keto philosophy. Some strict keto dieters will exclude fruit from their pantries all together because of this.

When it comes to non-starchy vegetables, there is a seemingly endless supply of options. The usual suspects are leafy greens like kale, spinach, various types of lettuce, so called "beet greens", arugula and chard. Then come your veggies belonging to the cruciferous family. These are your cauliflowers, broccolis, cabbage and Brussels sprouts. Also included in the non-starchy vegetable list are several types of squash, cucumbers, zucchini and asparagus. Green beans while technically a legume, also get lumped in this list because they have lower carbs than most legumes. Mung beans and mung bean shoots are also allowed because of low carbs. Non-starchy veggies from foreign cuisine like bolk choy are also allowed. Finally there are shoots and roots like carrots, celery, fennel, bamboo shoots and lemongrass. Other keto favorites include tomatoes, bell peppers, mushca amazing foods could have their own little section dedicated in this book listing their nutritional content and health benefits. All of these are considered whole foods, and you simply can't go wrong with them.

The ideal keto pantry will come stocked with a combination of leafy greens, cruciferous vegetables, tomatoes, bell peppers, garlic, onion and your choice of root, shoot, and type of squash.

There is no limit to the type of dishes you can make using these ingredients. You can mix and match, sauté, bake, stuff, broil, slice and simmer your way to keto excellence. Put a bunch of these ingredients in a pot and make a keto friendly stew, or heat up a pan with olive oil for a veggie sauté that can be eaten as is or as a side dish. The possibilities are endless.

Picking the Right Fats

Fat really isn't as unhealthy as it has been set it to be. The association between cardiovascular risk and cholesterol has been contested in recent years. The new universal killer is sugar and refined carbohydrates. And even if they don't kill, they bloat waistlines and make people feel miserable. There is nothing unhealthy about eating a diet that is more than half of fat—given that these fats are carefully chosen to provide the most benefit.

Fats in the keto diet generally come from three types. Saturated fat, monounsaturated fat, and polyunsaturated fats. Saturated fats are solid at room temperature and include things like butter and lard. Monounsaturated fats include avocados and olive oil. Polyunsaturated fats are the ones you find in fish oil and organic eggs. Meat can contain different types of fat depending on how it was sources. Grass fed beef, for example contains polyunsaturated fat as well as saturated fat.

Many will shudder at the mention of saturated fat, but it really isn't that bad for you. Its role in cardiovascular disease has been blown out of proportion since the war on fat took over the past half century.

Fat is used in the keto diet from everywhere. It is used to cook, to season, as a side, as a snack and even as the main course. Eating enough fat to fit the macro distribution in your diet really isn't that difficult once you consider that fat can be put on virtually anything and eaten with anything you wish. Keto recipes sometimes require a fatty oil as the base of the dish, which you will use for cooking. Olive oil dominates in this category, but other fats like butter, coconut oil, and ghee are also used from time to time. Whichever one you pick is more of a personal choice. Many go with an extra-virgin olive oil because it is universally used in many recipes and boasts a wide range of health benefits.

Avocados are a staple snack food and can be put on just about anything. They contain monounsaturated fats and are another one of those "super foods" that have emerged in recent years. You really can't go wrong with eating a few avocados in your diet. They are very low in carbs, so you can rack up the calories with them. Another viable monounsaturated fat are nuts such as almonds, pecans, chestnuts, and macadamias. Though be careful with raw nuts, they tend to be a little high in carbs. Try to avoid roasted varieties, and stick with plain.

Omega-6 is a polyunsaturated fat that is found in many food items, including meat. Most of us have a high ratio of omega-6 to omega-3, which presents a cardiovascular risk. Thankfully, keto can help create balance between the two. Omega-3's include fish with high fat content like salmon, eggs, and various seeds and nuts. All types of dairy are fair game (unless you are lactose intolerant). Milk however, even the whole fat variety, is high in carbs. You can quickly hit your max with a milk smoothie. Skim milks are reduces milks have even more carbs and are best avoided.

Fats to Avoid

Not all fats are created equal, and not all are allowed on keto. Fats you want to stay away from include refined vegetable oils that you might be used to cooking with. These are your canola, sunflower, corn and soybean oils.

By extension, avoid products that are made with any of these. Trans fats are also bad, and are found in margarine, cooking sprays and other spreads (Crisco).

Example Pantry List

Meat

- Chuck Roast
- Salmon
- Ground Beef (lean)
- Chicken Breast (With skin)
- Eggs
- Chicken thighs (with skin)
- Drumsticks
- Pork shoulder
- Canned Tuna
- Bacon Strips (unsweetened)
- Sirloin steak

Vegetables and Fruits

- Frozen berry mix
- Fresh blueberries
- Frozen chopped broccoli heads
- Baby Spinach
- Baby Carrots
- Small gala apples
- Celery Stalks

- Portobello Mushrooms (whole or sliced okay)
- Onion
- Summer Squash
- Bell Pepper (assorted)
- Tomatoes
- Kale
- Romaine Lettuce

Fats

- Extra-virgin olive oil
- Heavy Butter
- Your choice of cheese (mozzarella ,provolone, ricotta, etc)
- Almonds (raw)
- Coconut oil
- Avocados
- MCT oil
- Nut Butter
- Regular Butter
- Olives
- Full fat yogurt

Example Meal Plan

Monday

- Breakfast platter of hard boiled eggs, avocado slices and bacon strips

- Your choice of hot beverage (coffee ,tea, chai) with your choice of added fat (coconut oil, butter, MCT oil or mixture)
- Tuna wraps
- Salmon sautéed on olive oil for dinner, side of leafy greens
- Almonds for Snack

Tuesday

- Scrambled eggs, avocado and slices of tomato
- Hot beverage with fat added
- Bell pepper cheese melts
- Pulled chuck roast with side of baby carrots and peppers
- Fresh cheese for snack

Wednesday

- Small portion of smoked salmon with leafy greens
- Mixed berry shake (blended, add protein powder if desired)
- Chicken drum stick with a fatty dip (home made mayo, heavy cream)
- Left over pulled chuck

Thursday

- Egg omelet using your choice of spices and veggies
- Hot beverage with fat added
- Caesar salad with chicken breast strips or sirloin steak
- Shrimp and Bacon chowder

- Half avocado snack

Friday

- Bacon and egg frittata
- Kale and spinach shake
- Stove top chicken casserole
- Easy coconut oil fat bombs
- Tuna Salad

Saturday

- Sunny side up eggs with mix of veggies
- Hot beverage with fat added
- Meatball stew using ground beef, carrots, cabbage
- Baby carrots and fatty dip
- Berry and nut mix

Sunday

- Keto pancakes using eggs and almond flour
- Hot beverage with fat added
- Pork shoulder chops with side of greens
- shrimp skewers
- Your choice of keto fat bomb

CHAPTER 6:

Intermittent Fasting

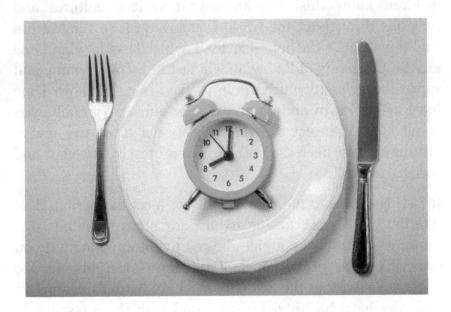

W hile not strictly part of the keto philosophy, its becoming more and more prevalent to use intermittent fasting and keto dieting together. Both techniques serve a similar purpose: to reverse the effects of sugar toxicity. Keto does it by switching the metabolic pathway from a glucose based one to fat based. Intermittent fasting does it by depriving the body from any exogenous caloric energy for a certain amount of time. In the weight loss triad mentioned in the previous chapter, intermittent fasting covers the topic of meal frequency.

At first glance, intermittent fasting sounds like one of the biggest fads out there. What does it even mean? Who are the fitness nerds who decided to put the word "intermittent" in front of it, and for what reason? Everyone knows what fasting is. We learn that bears eat large quantities of food during the window before fasting or going into hibernation. Even young children know this. We know that various cultures and religions throughout the world regularly fast. In the Muslim tradition there is the holy Ramadan, which lasts for about one month. Observers of Ramadan will fast in between sunup and sundown, for pretty much the entire day. They are allowed one meal before dawn and one meal after sunset. Typically, you aren't allowed to eat or drink in between those two meals. Fasting has also been used as a form of protest by prisoners and social activists.

If fasting means to not eat or drink for a certain period, then intermittent fasting means to fast for shorter periods. On intermittent fasts you aren't allowed to eat anything but you can drink water. In fact, constant hydration is recommended to offset the effects of the fast. Dry fasts are harder to complete and may have health risks associated with them (especially longer fasts). Intermittent fasting evolved from early calorie restriction diets and scientific studies that showed weight loss being associated with not eating. Obviously, somebody who stops receiving any nourishment will not be able to maintain body weight.

Intermittent fasting aims to use this weight loss factor and control it to for the dieters benefit. And like keto, it has been branded as a fringe, and even dangerous practice that shouldn't be taken lightly. On online forums people boast about their 3 three and week long fasts, which some individuals going for a month at a time of not eating. It is these extreme fasts that give intermittent fasting a bad name. Who are the people trying to test their own biology against the inevitable and why are they doing it? What do they hope to gain by not eating for a week or longer? Is going on a fast for that long even healthy? Is it sustainable?

When it comes to anecdotal evidence of this sort one must ask if such accounts are trustworthy. Going for just one day without eating is difficult enough. Some people can't even go a few hours without losing their senses. We also know that the human body needs some base form of nutrition to survive for long periods of famine. Electrolytes will fall perceptibly without any form of nutritional balance. So will other essential vitamins and minerals. Any one who goes a few days without eating is surely supplementing themselves with zero calorie substances—maybe a multivitamin or mineral water high in electrolytes. They are probably drinking water regularly. Dehydration will kill someone much earlier than starvation.

In truth, intermittent fasting has little to do with week long and month long fasts. Intermittent means periodically, on and off. For some this can mean fasting one day and eating normally on the next. Others fast everyday, but only few a few hours. It can be as simple as skipping breakfast everyday or having a late dinner. Whatever the case, they are doing it on the basis that it can help them lose weight. If no calories are coming in, then only calories are coming out. And with intermittent fasting you don't have to particularly watch what your eat or walk a certain amount of steps each day.

Starvation or Diet?

A traditional caloric restriction diet is one where you eat lower calories than what you burn. This can be a calculated difference, or something you can eyeball. If a standard diet consists of 2,000 calories a day, you would aim for a 1,800, 1,500 or 1,000 calorie diet. The logic is that eating less than you burn will cause your body to burn stored fat to make up for the deficit.

The problem here is that starvation doesn't quite work like that. The rate at which you burn calories depends on a several different factors and is never fixed. One day you might burn 2,200, and only burn 1,900 the next. It has to do with temperature regulation, activity level, and even on the thermal energy of the food you consume. What's more, it is dependent on the calories that you eat. Eat less calories and your body will naturally burn less. Eat more calories and your body will burn more. Why? Because your body is smart enough to try to preserve itself in times of famine or in our case, perceived famine. All body functions that require caloric energy but that are not essential for life are temporarily shut down because of the caloric deficit. This makes calorie restriction for weight loss somewhat of a toss up. It may work for you or it may not.

But intermittent fasting is different. Instead of getting some calories in by way of caloric restriction, you get absolutely zero. This in turn forces the body into the opposite of starvation mode—it goes into fat burning mode. With normal starvation conditions your body may be receiving a teeny bit of caloric energy, telling it to save what little it can get. It does this buy shutting off non-vital function. But if it doesn't receive any calories as is the case with intermittent fasting, it ramps up calorie expenditure instead. It sounds counterintuitive, but since our body prefers to use glucose, it will stop at nothing to find it. First it burns through available glucose store in the form of glycogen, the fast acting intermediary in between glucose and stored fat. Untapped glycogen stores will typically last between 24 and 36 hours. If a source of glucose hasn't been found, the body will then force itself to go into ketosis. Otherwise we would die. Thankfully most of us have ample fat stores to go around and keep us going.

Intermittent fasting is neither a diet nor is it starvation. It isn't a diet because you aren't eating anything like how you would with a calorie restriction diet. It isn't starvation because you aren't really starving. What you are doing is using the same mechanisms of starvation to help you burn extra fat. Its not an eating disorder either. Intermittent fasting is completely healthy, and fasting has been used by many peoples across the world for spiritual and religious purposes. If fasting was inherently dangerous, it wouldn't be so popular with the Muslims, Buddhists, Christians and several others that regularly partake in it. We also wouldn't have made it this far as a species. We would have all died for starvation long ago.

How to Get Started Fasting

In short, one could fast by simply skipping one or two meals. The same mechanisms behind starvation survival begin to kick in as soon as the body requires more energy and can't find it. But intermittent fasting becomes more regular than simply skipping one or two meals. It should ideally be done on a routine of either an alternating day basis or daily. Longer fasts can be done once or twice a week. There are many different intermittent fasting schemes that you can use. Whichever one you choose will depend on your lifestyle. Some people prefer to skip breakfast, for example. Others don't like eating after dark. As with diet, your lifestyle and fasting habits need to be in perfect harmony to maximize success.

Twelve Hour Fast

For somebody just starting out, a 12 hour fasting scheme is one of the easiest to employ. At first it sounds a little difficult, but everyone already fasts for about 8 hours (hopefully!) when they are asleep. This time carries over to the total time spent fasting. The conditions under sleep are not much different from the conditions being awake, metabolically speaking. You will burn slightly fewer calories while asleep but over eight hours the fat burning opportunities compound. Following sleep, you will fast for another four hours. Meaning that you can only drink water or other zero calorie drinks like coffee and tea. For obvious reasons, sugary drinks are out of the question. Anything you wouldn't drink on keto you shouldn't drink on the fast. Mineral water, seltzer and other forms of carbonated waters are fine.

For maximum efficiency, you can choose what twelve hours you will fast. If you eat your last meal around mid afternoon, you should be able to enjoy breakfast the next morning and still be fasted for twelve hours. Alternatively you can eat your last meal later in the day, and have a late lunch to break the fast.

Generally, the twelve hour fast can be done daily or on an alternating day basis. Don't worry too much about counting calories at this stage. The time restriction of intermittent fasting will force you to eat less anyways. At the same time, make sure you follow your keto diet to the letter. If you eat a carby meal and get out of ketosis, your fasting would be for nothing.

16/8 Fast

Similar to the 12 hour fast, but with a longer fasting time. With the 16/8 fast your can eat during a period of eight hours and fast for the other 16. Since the eating window is quite small, you might prefer to eat two large meals instead of the standard three. You should eat filling proteins at each meal so that you don't get hungry as much. And since the fasting period is so long, you probably will get hungry sometime after having your last meal. Again, you are free to chose which sixteen hours you fast for and time spent sleeping counts.

The 16/8 fast can easily be modified to become more difficult. Simply add time to the fasting duration and take away from the eating window. Fasts that are 18/6, and 20/4 are possible. You can do the 16/8 fast daily or on an alternating basis.

24 Hour Fast

Fasting for an entire day blurs the line between intermittent fasting and a regular fast. Twenty four hours is a long time—you won't be able to eat anything until the next day. It also requires increased willpower to successfully pull off. Few of us can imagine spending an entire eight hours at work and then come home to a completely empty stomach. You should ideally do a few 12 hour and 16/8 fasts beforehand, periodically increasing the fasting duration so that you get used to longer fasts. Obviously, you won't be able to go on this fast everyday. Even alternate day fasting with this one may be too much. Listen to what your body tells you. People who use this fast prefer to do it twice a week, and preferably no more than three.

Beyond 36 Hours

In non keto acclimatized people, the 36 hour mark will be around the time that glycogen stores get all used up. If they aren't already in ketosis, their body will slowly start making the transition. Glycogen stores can normally store around 1,800 to 2,000 calories, but not much more than that. Fat in the form of adipose tissue on the other hand, has no limit to stored calories. For this reason the body has a natural preference for the order in which fuel is burned. First is glucose, then glycogen and finally fat. Sometimes protein gets stuck in the mix, and will be used for fuel around the glycogen mark before ketosis kicks in. Note that it is possible to lose lean body mass in this manner when going on a longer (24 hours or more) fast. If you want to lose weight but retain muscle mass, these longer fasts may not be suitable for you.

Going for this long without consuming any nutrients will begin to take its toll on you. Make sure you supplement your electrolyte balance as well as take a daily multivitamin. Two 36 hour fasts a week is about how much you want to do. Any more would be asking for trouble.

Fasts beyond 36 hours are usually only recommended for people who are very overweight or obese. These people stand to benefit the most, and fasts that last multiple days are suitable for them. The possibility of losing lean muscle mass is a considerable risk, one that should be factored into your weight loss goals. One can expect to lose about 1/3 of a pound per day of lean body mass while water fasting. This means that a three day fast will effectively cost you 1 lbs of lean body mass (most of this will be in the form of muscle weight). For the average person trying to lose weight, a 36 hour fast should be treated as a hard upper limit.

Protein Sparing Modified Fast

What if told you that you could reap most of the benefits of water fasting, minus the loss in lean muscle mass? Such a thing is possible using a protein sparing modified fast (PSMF), but it really isn't a fast in the sense that a water fast is a fast. With a water fast you are not allowed to consume calories at all, but with PSMF you can. Still, you will limit your calories to 800 to 1,000 a day, and no lower than 600. With this daily calorie requirement it is more akin to a calorie restriction diet. PSMF was popularized by physicians in the 1970's to treat morbidly obese patients. The PSMF traditionally consisted a strict diet that allowed for 1.2 grams of protein per the desired goal weight for the patient. If the goal weight was 180, for example, the patient was allowed 218 grams of protein, which may sound like a lot, but it only ends up being 864 calories. Patients were also allowed some 20g – 50g of carbohydrates and no additional fats. This low-carb requirement is similar to the standard keto diet as you may no doubt recognize it. This version of the PSMF was used mostly in a clinical setting with heavy supervision of patients. It typically lasted a few weeks to 6 months. After those six months, the patient was gradually reintroduced to more carbohydrates and fats. In short, to a regular standard diet in time. But they would have dropped several pounds of fat from the calorie restriction based diet, and suffered minimal losses in lean body mass. They can lose up to 40 pounds of mostly fat in a 12 week period.

The most striking difference between PSMF and a regular intermittent fast is the duration. For best results, a PSMF should last between 6 and 12 weeks, in which you can see weight loss of 2 lbs a week or more (especially during the first few weeks). If you decide to go on PSMF, make sure you are already keto acclimatized before startin. This will ensure that your body is in tip top fat burning shape. The meals you eat during your PSMF will typically be the same as the ones on keto, with the exception of fat. Keto recipes often require you to go out of your way to use fats in your cooking and as additives to the main dish. If you do use fat to cook your meals on PSMF, use only the bare minimum for seasoning and frying. A few dashes of olive oil probably won't interfere with your fast.

Fasting Tips

As you may have guessed, fasting is not an easy endeavor. Like with the beginning of keto, you will have to get used to the effects of a lengthy fast. If your body isn't used to it, fasting will definitely cause you some pain. On your fasting days you can expect hunger pangs, headaches, and general feelings of lethargy. The brunt of these bothersome symptoms will have to do with the affects of low blood sugar. For people who are already in ketosis, this presents less of a problem. You can still expect to feel hunger and general feelings of irritability, but it will be much bearable. This is why it is highly recommended to first get into ketosis by restricting carbohydrates than to force ketosis by going on a fast. Both fasting and a regular low-carb diet will ultimately compliment each other. Using both will maximize fat burning capabilities. First, the keto diet pumps triglycerides directly to a metabolic pathway primed for using fat as energy. Then, the fast take cares of pesky body fat you have stored.

There is no easy way to make a fast enjoyable. The key is to keep yourself busy throughout the day and to eliminate situations that trigger your cravings (either for fat or sugar). Make sure you drink plenty of water. Feel free to hydrate more than you would normally do. If you are used to drinking 2 liters of water a day, try doing 2.5, 3 or even one gallon a water. You shouldn't fear gaining water weight by doing this. Most of our water weight comes from glycogen stores which tend to absorb large quantities of it. Drinking up to a gallon of water a day will be negligible for water weight if your are already in ketosis. Whenever you feel a hunger pang coming, drown your cravings with a nice cool glass of water. Remember that you can drink other zero calorie substances as well, like tea and coffee. Other commercial products that contain "zero calories" are not recommended, as they probably contain some artificial sweetener. Diet soda is an absolute no, but you may wish to buy electrolyte infused drinks (as long as they have minimal artificial sweeteners).

Part of staying busy means avoiding situations where food may be involved. This includes skipping on lunch outings with coworkers, avoiding areas like kitchens, cafeterias and food courts when outside of the house. When you are in your residence, try to hide food that is easily accessible. Don't leave snacks laying around the kitchen, living room or bedroom.

Diabetics and people with other medication conditions should be extremely exercise caution when going on a fast. Some level of medical supervision is preferred, and medical clearance by a doctor or qualified physician is required. Diabetes are more likely to suffer a life threatening instance of low blood sugar if they skip too many meals, especially when taking insulin medications. If at any time a diabetic feels faint, or experiences gaps in consciences, they should immediately stop the fast.

Other wise healthy individuals should stop a fast when severe symptoms of vomiting or diarrhea are present. Fairing, feeling lightheaded or losing consciousness in any other form is also grounds for stopping a fast. Regular hydration and replenishing of electrolytes may alleviate some of these symptoms, but if everything else fails, it is time to eat something.

Always break a fast with a small meal or snack. Then allow for thirty minutes or so to eat a major meal. You do not want to flood your system will food all at once. It could make you sick or upset your stomach. Typically this meal should be no more than 500 calories.

Finally, plan your fasts around major social events and other outings were food is a major topic. Avoid telling all your friends about your fasting habits and look for a core group of supporters who will coexist with your eating habits. These can be a roommate or significant other that you live with. Ultimately, the people you are closest with or see everyday will be most affected by your fasting routines. You don't have to convince them to fast alongside you, but they should be able to give you the space that you need and respect your health decisions.

Do I Have to Fast? If Not, Why Should I do it?

If you feel like fasting isn't for you, there isn't any pressure to do so. You can still lose weight in healthy, controlled increments by using the keto diet alone.

However, if you are looking for a rapid weight loss solution, fasting on top of keto is a sure fire way to do it. Fasting, when done correctly, is perfectly safe. Some version of intermittent fasting, straight fasting, or PSMF diets are prescribed to obese patients all the time.

If you still aren't convinced, its no big deal. But there are plenty of other reasons why you may wish to go on a fast every once a while. Its a way of being good to your body by letting it rest from the constant cycle of caloric absorption.

Though to us digestion seems perfectly fine, it causes our bodies a great deal of stress. Just think, if our brains could transmit pain signals throughout the whole digestion process, we would probably never eat again. But since it is a vital human function, our brains have learned to block out these signals over time.

Think about all of the inflammation and mechanical forces that go into turning solid foods into nutrients.

Fasting has another magical property that has to do with movements at the cellular level. Depriving cells of nutrients encourage them to repair broken down cellular building blocks and repurpose them, instead of waiting for more from food. This is a mechanism called autophagy, it can be triggered by going on a fast that lasts 12-16 hours or more. Autophagy may even reduce wrinkled skin, as cells decide to do away with old cellular gunk that we no longer need.

Autophagy is an excellent companion after drastic weight loss for getting your skin feeling tight again. It can also slow down the aging process, as autophagy natural slows down with age. Inducing it by going on a medium to long fast ignores the factor of an aging body that wont induce autophagy on its own.

CHAPTER 7:

Keto And Exercise

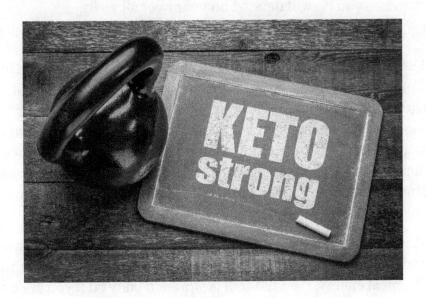

The final major component in the weight loss triad is exercise. We have all heard it before, sometimes to the point of exhaustion, but exercise serves a valuable purpose. Even when diet gets lauded as being responsible for 95% of all weight loss, exercise may still help you burn extra fat, feel better about yourself, and raise metabolism. These are all good, healthy goals that everyone should strive to achieve through regular physical activity. Exercising on keto has some caveats, but is completely safe. In fact, many athletes prefer to work out when they are in full ketosis mode rather than stick to the same old carbohydrate loading and crashing cycle.

Both aerobic and anaerobic exercise should be used. People who want to build muscle and lose fat should opt for more anaerobic, and people who want to burn more fat should do more aerobics. In other words, lift heavy weights for the combined benefit of muscle growth and greater metabolism, and walk, run or jog to burn off additional fat. Which types of exercises you do will depend on your over all goals.

Exercise and the Ketogenic Lifestyle

There are many benefits to exercising while being on the keto diet. First, you are able to push yourself to greater limits without succumbing to carbohydrate crashes. You also directly use fat for an energy source, thereby skipping the intermediary step of first wasting glucose and glycogen stores and then burning fat. Ultimately, no keto lifestyle is as complete or as effective as one that includes a healthy mix of aerobic and anaerobic activity.

Moving your body helps circulate blood, raises your heart rate and contracts the muscles. There are actions that require chemical energy, the kind that is stored in body fat if you are on ketosis. They also make you a healthier person overall. Blood moving through your veins helps lower inflammation and dilates the blood vessels, helping you fight cardiovascular disease over time. Exercise is especially important for those with desk jobs who do a lot of sitting.

Exercise under the ketogenic lifestyle is little different from exercise on any other diet. The activity recommendations for children and adults is the same. At the very minimum, it is recommended to get 150 minutes of aerobic exercise a week. This can be split up between low intensity work, like walking and high intensity workouts like HIT and CrossFit. Strength training is recommended for three sessions each week each week using moderate to light weight if weight loss is the goal.

The only major difference is exercising on a fast. You may feel less energy (if not in fully ketosis) and hence you might justify skipping a workout because you haven't eaten that day. This is largely a misconception. The average person will be able to workout just as fine on a fast. Diabetics and others need to approach exercise with care. And this again has to do with low blood sugar counts. It is not recommended that a diabetic exercise during a fast if their blood sugar is too low.

Using Exercise to Tip the Fat Burning Scale

The amount of fat your body burns on keto will still depend on your daily BMR. To maximize fat burning, then, you need to create an energetic deficit by doing moderate to intense exercise. Simply following the recommended exercise guidelines may be enough for most people. Those seeking to get the most out of their diet and exercise routine should exercise more regularly. Instead of 150 minutes, 300 or 450 minutes a week is ideal. The best type of exercise for burning fat is, you guessed it, cardio. Running, walking, Stairmaster, spin classes and Pilates are all good options. Throw in a 2 to 3 weightlifting sessions a week and you will also boost natural fat burning through muscle synthesis and greater metabolism.

But exercise doesn't have to end in the gym or walking trail. It is trivial to increase daily calories expended by simply moving more around the house or workplace. Consider biking to work ever so often or taking public transportation (if your city is amendable to these things). The distance you walk from the bust stop can add up over time. Simply do more things. Clean up around your house even if nothing needs to be cleaned. Get up from your chair every hour. Sneak in breaks to do push ups or body weight squats in the bathroom. Do whatever it takes to tip the fat burning scale into your favor.

Is Working Out In Ketosis Safe?

Unless you are diabetic or have some other medical concern, it is safe to exercise with your body in full ketosis. In fact, you might find that it is much easier to do so. Your energetic output will be much higher than if you were on a standard diet. If you are fasting, try to time your workouts within your eating window or at the tail end of your fasting period. This way you can immediately refuel after a workout, and give your muscles the protein and other nutrients they need.

CHAPTER 8:

Weight Loss Check List and Keto FAQ

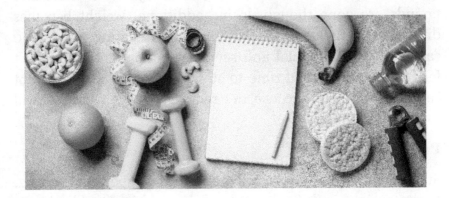

You may find that you lose weight quickly on keto but then the results taper off. Most of the weight you lose in the beginning will be from water weight, as your excess glycogen stores release trapped water. There really isn't anything to fear with weight loss plateau's because they are expected, even on the keto diet. A prolonged plateau that lasts weeks may simply indicate that the energetic balance in your body has peaked—you won't be able to lose anymore weight unless you bring down calories or increase the frequency of fasting.

Ask yourself what your goal was in the first place. If you find that you still have more pounds to go and you haven't reached your goal yet, a plateau can be worrying. It still doesn't have to mean that the diet has failed you, or that you don't stand to benefit from having a keto lifestyle. Something else could be going wrong with your approach. For these cases, there is a small checklist you might want to go through to see where the issue lies.

Eating Too Much

As with any diet, an excess of calories will make it difficult to lose weight. Even on keto you can expect to lose some pounds while eating more or less the same as always. After these first pounds are gone though, losing additional weight becomes difficult with the same caloric surplus. Try eating 200 – 300 calories less than usual and see what happens. If you aren't fasting, now is a good time to start. You don't have to count calories as much, because the reduced eating windows will force you to eat less.

Point of Stagnation

Stagnation in your diet can be due to improper goal setting. Losing weight is difficult, and requires a fair bit of patience. Normally what we call fat is measured by taking the body mass index. There are several ways to do this, but the easiest is to use the caliper test, for which there are many conversion tables available.

The following table is based off Accu-Measure brand calipers for determining body fat. It is compatible with both sexes.

Accu-Measure Reading in Millimeters

AGE	2-3	4-5	6-7	8-9	10-11	12-13	14-15	16-17	18-19	20-21	22-23	24-25	26-27	28-29	30-31	32-33	34-36
18-20	2.0	3.9	6.2	8.5	10.5	12.5	14.3	16.0	17.5	18.9	20.2	21.3	22.3	23.1	23.8	24.3	24.9
21-25	2.5	4.9	7.3	9.5	11.6	13.6	15.4	17.0	18.6	20.0	21.2	22.3	23.3	24.2	24.9	25.4	25.8
26-30	3.5	6.0	8.4	10.6	12.7	14.6	16.4	18.1	19.6	21.0	22.3	23.4	24.4	25.2	25.9	26.5	26.9
31-35	4.5	7.1	9.4	11.7	13.7	15.7	17.5	19.2	20.7	22.1	23.4	24.5	25.5	26.3	27.0	27.5	28.0
36-40	5.6	8.1	10.5	12.7	14.8	16.8	18.6	20.2	21.8	23.2	24.4	25.6	26.5	27.4	28.1	28.6	29.0
41-45	6.7	9.2	11.5	13.8	15.9	17.8	19.6	21.3	22.8	24.7	25.5	26.6	27.6	28.4	29.1	29.7	30.1
46-50	7.7	10.2	12.6	14.8	16.9	18.9	20.7	22.4	23.9	25.3	26.6	27.7	28.7	29.5	30.2	30.7	31.2
51-55	8.8	11.3	13.7	15.9	18.0	20.0	21.8	23.4	25.0	26.4	27.6	28.7	29.7	30.6	31.2	31.8	32.2
56 & UP	9.9	12.4	14.7	17.0	19.1	21.0	22.8	24.5	26.0	27.4	28.7	29.8	30.8	31.6	32.3	32.9	33.3

LEAN   IDEAL   AVERAGE   ABOVE AVERAGE

Someone who lies on the above average category should strive to get their weight to the average, or ideal category. People who are already in the ideal or average range will have a harder time losing weight. If you belong to this group, don't be too hard on yourself if you aren't reaching your weight loss goals right away. It takes time and effort.

Not Eating a Clean Diet

The stricter the keto diet the better. Your results will very much depend on the foods that you are eating. In particular, watch out for artificial sweeteners and other places that sugar might sneak in. Not counting daily carbs is good way to excuse "cheat meals" that you may be eating without realizing. The goal is to stay in ketosis for as long as possible, and eating too much carbs simply won't do.

You may be eating something that you thought was keto, or that someone made you believe it was keto when in reality it contained carbs or sugar. This is particularly dangerous with online communities. When in doubt, look the food up. Large databases of virtually every type of food are available online which can tell you the exact carbohydrate content of each food.

Not Getting Enough Exercise

You can blame your diet for not giving you faster results, or you can take matters into your own hand and tip the fat burning scale. Adequate aerobic and anaerobic exercise will help you burn extra calories when it is needed. If you are having a hard time burning additional fat after several weeks on the diet, you might consider starting a resistance training routine. The extra muscle you build will give your metabolism a boost, raise lean body mass, and ultimately burn more fat in the long run.

Not Getting Enough Sleep

Recovery time is important, both for you mind and body. Fasting gives you a break from digestion, and sleeping gives you a break from the stresses of everyday life. Do not skimp on sleep. It is an important processes were cells repair themselves and recycled unused resources. You should aim for 7 - 8 hours of sleep every night

Keto FAQ, Final Tips and Tricks

How do I stay motivated on the diet?

Keto isn't easy, and neither is finding the motivation to do it. Over time though you will become more used to eating fat instead of carbs.

Ask yourself what the true source of motivational change comes from. Is it that you miss bread and other carbs? Are you tired of cooking keto recipes vs going out to eat? You don't have to go all out with your meals, many simple recipes exist. Do not underestimate the power of leftovers. You will find that most keto recipes call for 2 – 4 servings or more. Many of these can easily be reheated for a quick dinner.

Is Keto worth it?

It certainly is. Giving up certain foods doesn't mean you must give up taste.

Plenty of keto meals are delicious as they are filling. Alternatives for many popular foods like pizza and pasta are also available. Your body and your liver will thank you for making the switch

What does it mean when you say that certain people need medical supervision?

In short, it means having some correspondence with a doctor or primary care physician. It doesn't have to be constant surveillance like with scientific studies, but somebody in charge of your health should definitely know what you are doing.

Is keto expensive?

Keto doesn't have to cost anymore than what a standard diet does. Take away the frequent meals eaten at resultants and fast food places and the price tapers off. Some food like organic and grass fed will cost more—but are not necessary for the diet. Meat in general is expensive yes, but most of your calories are coming from fat, not meat. Cheaper cuts of meat are always available as well. Fats, in general, aren't too expensive food.

What other health concerns exist, if any?

Other than the ones covered, virtually none. Cholesterol may be an issue, and is the most commonly cited health concern. But if you are using the good fats, and a healthy ratio of omega-3 and omega-6, there is little to worry about

Who Recommends Keto?

There is a growing body of physicians, health commentators and fitness experts who are standing by the diet. Low-carb diets have always been used to treat diabetes and obesity. Proponents of keto like Dr. Jason Fung have done extensive research on its ability to reverse type 2 diabetes and fight obesity.

What are the common keto mistakes?

Eating too much, continuing to eat out at restaurants without doing any research on the meals, and eating the wrong stuff. Keto uses easy concepts, but they are harder to implement in real life. There are also too many processed foods on the market that advertise themselves as keto. Just because something is low-carb, it doesn't automatically make it keto friendly. The whole foods aspect also needs to considered.

Another common mistake is letting social pressure disrupt the diet. Your friends and family may be critical of your new diet and try to dissuade you from following it. But if you are reaching your goals, then what is the point of their criticism? You have to ignore them, even if means losing a few friendships. Instead, look for those who want to support you and elevate your actions.

Finally, letting others dictate your eating habits by way of social influence. Eating is a powerful social activity that is used during celebrations and holidays. Since holidays are rare, it is okay to break your diet on these special occasions. But if someone is inviting you to eat constantly, it is time to put your foot down on the matter and say no.

CHAPTER 9:

Recipes

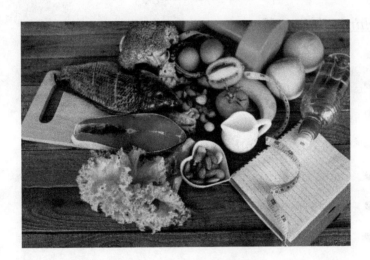

Keto recipes come in many shapes and sizes. Some are simple, and others complex. Let's face it—there's only so many ways that you can prepare the same chicken, beef, salmon and eggs. Keto recipes that are simple are always the best because you can expand on them however you like. Swap out ingredients here, add something there. With keto you want to always be adding fat wherever you can. Whether that means using a different type of oil, or preparing a side dish to go with the main course is up to you. There are countless ways to prepare keto friendly versions of common food additives. Keto mayonnaise, dips, salad dressing and meat marinade are all possible. As always, remind yourself that your cooking should reflect the diet. No spurious adding of sugar here, or using carboy ingredients. If you look hard enough for alternatives, you can usually find a keto friendly version. Using almond flour, for example, opens up a new realm of possible for baked goods esque cuisine. All without the worry of eating too many carbs.

Here are some easy to follow example recipes that you can experiment with and alter accordingly.

Zucchini Mini Muffins

- 1 tsp baking powder
- 1 tsp baking soda
- 3 eggs
- 1 ½ cup almond flour
- 1 cup zucchini (grated)
- 1 tbs ground cinnamon
- 1 tsp vanilla extract
- ¼ cup coconut oil

1. To start, preheat oven to 350 degrees
2. Finely Grate the zucchini
3. Combine eggs, vanilla extract and coconut oil
4. Add the contents of bowl into rest of ingredients
5. Lastly add the grated zucchini into bowl mixture
6. Use coconut oil to grease muffin pan wells
7. Add the mixture to each well and bake for 10 – 12 minutes
8. Let cool and enjoy

Spinach Frittata

- 3 oz pancetta or bacon strips
- 2 cup thinly grated carrots
- 2 cups baby spinach leaves
- salt and pepper or other seasoning
- 3 – 6 eggs (depending on preferred portion size)
- ½ cup onion diced
- 1/3 cup coconut milk (all natural)

1. Whisk eggs in mixing bowl
2. Add the coconut milk and whatever seasonings you like
3. Set oven to 350 degrees
4. Gently brown pancetta or bacon with medium heat. Leave fat on frying pan Make sure pan is oven safe. Remove pancetta or bacon
5. Cook onions and carrots with the leftover fat
6. Cook the spinach
7. Pour egg mixture on top of frying pan and let cook for 2 minutes
8. Sprinkle the bacon pancetta into cooked mixture
9. Place pan into oven and bake for 20 – 25 minutes

Shrimp and meatball skillet

- 8 oz ground beef, balled
- Olive oil
- 16 oz medium shrimp peeled
- 1 summer squash chopped
- ¾ Cup of sliced bell pepper
- ¼ Cup chicken broth (preferably home made)
- ½ onion
- Salt and pepper
- Your choice of additional seasonings (paprika, cumin, red pepper)

1. Prepare skillet or wok with olive oil
2. Add shrimp, ground beef balls and cook for few minutes. Set aside
3. Use 2 tbsp. olive oil to sauté onions and peppers
4. Add shrimp, meat balls and squash into skillet, cook for 2 minutes
5. Add chicken broth to moisten
6. Finally season with salt, pepper seasoning of your choice

Slow Cooked Pot Roast

- 2 Lbs chuck roast
- 8 oz mushrooms sliced
- 1 onion, diced
- 3 tbsp olive oil
- 3 tbsp tomato paste
- 2/3 cup beef broth
- Your choice of garnishes and spices
- 3 cloves of garlic
- Salt and pepper

1. Season chuck roast with salt and pepper
2. Sear chuck in a large skillet using olive oil. Lightly brown, do not cook fully for about 2-3 minutes
3. Place chuck roast in slow cooker, add onions, mushrooms and garlic gloves. Roast should go above
4. Add the broth and paste into the slow cooker
5. Add your choice of seasonings and spices (rosemary, thyme oregano, etc
6. Set slow cooker for six hours on high, or 8-12 hours on low.
7. Roast is ready when tender and easy to pull with fork

Keto Chicken Lettuce Wraps

- 1 lbs ground chicken or turkey
- 2 green onion chopped
- 1 butter lettuce head (or romaine)
- 1 cup chopped onion
- salt and pepper
- A fatty sauce to top it off (heavy cream, keto mayo, soy sauce
- olive oil

1. Heat up a skillet with olive oil to brown the chicken. Cook for 2 – 3 minutes
2. Add in onions, cook for 2 minutes using the same fat in the skillet
3. When ready to serve, pack chicken neatly into lettuce leaves. Add the fatty sauce or filling ant top off with green onions

Coconut Protein Balls

- ½ cup pitted dates
- 1 tsp vanilla extract
- 3 tbsp protein powder of choice
- ½ cup almond butter
- 2/3 cup shredded coconut
- 1/3 cup pecans halved

1. Puree dates with almond butter and vanilla extract in a blender
2. Add mixture into mixing bowl and mix in protein powder, half the shredded coconut and pecans
3. Use the remaining coconut to top off rolled balls of the mixture
4. Keep refrigerated

Conclusion

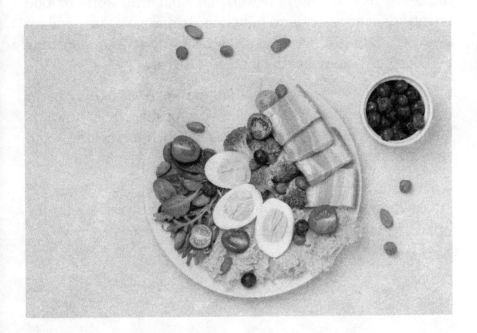

You now have everything that you need to begin on your ketogenic journey. Along the way you may learn new ways of doing things, new recipes and techniques for perfecting the keto lifestyle. This is not a final destination by any means. Keep an open mind as you approach new diets and learn more about the science behind ketosis.

Always be looking for new techniques to help you get where you need to get. Experiment with different exercise and fasting schemes until you find one that fits best. Your health is one of the most important things you have in this world, and it bears putting in the hard work.

Decide for yourself what is the best healthy lifestyle for you. Accept any and all criticism and be constantly in search for new information on old and tired dieting advice. Keto has opened the doors for many into the wild and wonderful world of food science, biochemistry and nutrition. It doesn't take a college degree to be an expert, or at least know what is happening between our bodies and the food that we eat.

This is valuable knowledge that everyone has to right to explore. Hopefully, this book was a positive step towards kindling new interest for the science behind healthy, and sustainable lifestyles.

Finally, make sure to leave a review if you found this information useful! And help spread the word about the wonders of the ketogenic diet.

CPSIA information can be obtained
at www.ICGtesting.com
Printed in the USA
BVHW061922220321
603177BV00010B/908